Keeping Busy

Keeping Busy

A Handbook of Activities for Persons with Dementia

James R. Dowling

The Johns Hopkins University Press
Baltimore and London

© 1995 The Johns Hopkins University Press
All rights reserved. Published 1995
Printed in the United States of America on acid-free paper
2 4 6 8 9 7 5 3

This book was prepared under the propriety of
Kennebec Long Term Care, Inc.

The Johns Hopkins University Press
2715 North Charles Street
Baltimore, Maryland 21218-4363
www.press.jhu.edu

Library of Congress Cataloging-in-Publication Data

Dowling, James R.
Keeping busy : a handbook of activities for persons with
dementia / James R. Dowling.
p.   cm.
Includes bibliographical references and index.
ISBN 0-8018-5058-4 (hc : alk. paper).—ISBN 0-8018-5059-2
(pbk. : alk. paper)
1. Alzheimer's disease—Patients—Rehabilitation.   2. Alzheimer's
disease —Patients—Recreation.   3. Occupational therapy for the aged.
4. Day care centers for the aged—Activity programs.
5. Nursing homes—Recreational activities.   I. Title.
[DNLM: 1. Alzheimer's Disease—rehabilitation.
2. Day Care—methods.   3. Long-Term Care—methods.
WM 220 D747k 1995]
RC523.D675   1995
616.8´3—dc20
DNLM/DLC for Library of Congress
94-42721

A catalog record for this book is available from the British Library.

Contents

Foreword

Alzheimer disease and many of the related disorders remain chronic diseases. We cannot cure them and can do little to halt their devastating impact. The dementias have a profound effect on the impaired person's life. Because they change the person's behavior, they affect the lives of all those around them as well.

The goal of a therapeutic activity program is to minimize the behavioral damage and sustain as long as possible the keys to personhood. Because the dementias have more than one victim, we also seek to normalize behaviors so that those around the impaired person—families, other residents, and staff—are also more comfortable.

A good activity program restores a sense of purpose, identity, and control. It enables old roles and makes familiar tasks possible. It helps an impaired person feel good about herself and enables her to enjoy other people. There is strong evidence that these positive experiences reduce many behavior problems.

The theory behind these activities has been described. However, families and care providers have found it difficult to implement activities with these outcomes. Many activity directors who make an effort to enhance their program still find some participants who are sleeping, some who are wandering, one or two who are shouting, and one who is absorbed in disassembling her soiled diaper—but few who join in a carefully planned activity or show evidence of being enriched by it.

Numerous articles and books (in particular, *Doing Things,* by Jitka Zgola, and *Dementia Care,* edited by Nancy Mace) describe the principles underlying good activity care for persons with dementia. But principles are not enough; Jim Dowling also shows us what to do and how. He not only clearly and simply conveys the concepts underlying activities for persons with dementia but also gives pages and pages of activities that work and describes in detail how to implement them. This will be invaluable to anyone responsible for an activity program.

One of the best-kept secrets in dementia care is that in good settings, caregiving is fun. Jim's own joy in the work he does is evident in his writing and is a breath of fresh air for the reader. This book gives an excellent example of how this staff works as a team and has integrated activities into all aspects of care. The activities are simple and do not require complicated or expensive supplies.

I visited the Alzheimer's Care Center, in Gardiner, Maine, where Jim works his magic. The residents are quite capable of serious outbursts of anger, but such problems are uncommon. (I spent my day flashing flashbulbs in their faces as I took photographs, and provoked only smiles and posing.) This cheery, homelike facility is filled with people who are amiable, participating, going places, doing things, keeping busy. The facility demonstrates that this activity program, as part of the total team effort, does work. Problem behaviors are minimized and the sense of self is retained. Smiles are common.

Keeping Busy is a hands-on, practical book written by an expert in activities and in dementia care. It is rich in compassion for those who are impaired, and it presents the skills needed to bring a few moments of joy to them.

Nancy L. Mace

Acknowledgments

For a period of time, I have considered myself to be uncommonly fortunate. I've been able to think, reflect, and write about a job that I love. It has been a very motivational and educational process.

I am deeply indebted to the following people for their assistance and expertise.

Marian Anderson, Professor of Music, Bates College. Birdie Katz, for her musical expertise and talent and for her abiding, specifically and generally. Robin Miller, who has served as our Arts Consultant, and has done so with fitting flexibility, insight, and wit.

Mary Plumer and Nancy Eames, Community Relations office, Kennebec Health Systems, for their advice and efforts.

Linette Miller and Marc Loiselle, for their phenomenally generous assistance and labor, expertise, and for the machines! Without their efforts, this book would never have found its way out of the wilderness.

Greg Gravel, Exec. V.P., K.L.T.C., for the faith and time to do the work.

Wendy Harris, of the Johns Hopkins University Press, for her patient, succinct, and friendly guidance, which helped the whole enterprise be a pleasant surprise.

Nancy Mace: trustworthy expert, fearless advocate, colleague, and friend.

Bea Dorbacker, for advice, encouragement, and perusal.

Larry Tibbetts: past president, National Remotivation Technique Organization; member, International Advisory Board; sounding board, confrere, and fellow traveler.

Above all, my co-workers, with whom I have learned the most, especially Marion Boynton, Laura Colomb, and Judy Stevens, who were there when the doors opened and are still there (and to Cyndie Heath, who wasn't but might as well have been). Elizabeth Burbeck, whose spirit is still with us. Debbie Madore, who helped us all appreciate the value of laughter. Dawn Thomas, who helped us appreciate the gifts of faith. Dixie Leavitt, who helped get both the center and the day care off the ground; Linda Vannah, who carried both far; and Mary Bailey, who has given the program new and beautiful wings. Special thanks to Vicki Christie, great learner and great teacher, for her careful scrutiny of the manuscript (and detailed comments); Jane O'Rourke, for being our soul and conscience; Mary Nicholas, the rock upon which we have grown; and Jessie Jacques, who made the whole thing possible and who has been both mother and father to the bunch of us.

I would finally like to acknowledge Jim and Nina Dowling, who showed a while back that aging, memory, and good humor can go hand in hand.

Prologue

Mollie was nervous. A few minutes earlier she had been calm. In a few minutes more, if left to her own devices, she would be frantic. She looked worried; she asked for help. As usual for her, the questions were, "Have you seen Bertha, my daughter?" and "Where did I leave my car?"

It was picnic day. Sandwich preparation was just getting under way in the kitchen. Mollie, always glad to help, was easily engaged in peeling and chopping hard-cooked eggs. Before long, attentive to her task, her anxiety melted and her normal good humor—her "calm state"—returned.

"You know," she said, glancing aside from her work, "this is good. Because time flies when you're . . ." Her hands froze in midmotion; her mouth was open, tongue poised to say the lost word, to complete the adage.

I prompted, "Time flies when you're . . ."

"Yes," she replied, smiling. "Time flies when you're busy." Her hands resumed their task. She added, "Then you don't get nervous."

Not trusting myself to remember the words or even the exchange, I wrote Mollie's words on a handy napkin. I lost the napkin, as it happened, but the episode had committed itself to memory.

$$\bullet \; {}^\bullet_\bullet \; \bullet$$

Introduction

This book is the outcome of a program of activities for persons with dementia, developed at the Alzheimer's Care Center in Gardiner, Maine. It is offered in the hope that other caregivers can benefit from and build on our experiences.

• The Alzheimer's Care Center •

The Facility

When the Alzheimer's Care Center (A.C.C.) opened in February 1988, it was the first freestanding, dementia-dedicated facility of its kind in the United States. It was designed to meet the needs of persons with Alzheimer disease and related dementias through innovative, non-medical techniques. The facility is small enough to be manageable, yet has enough space for individual activity and privacy. The design is intended to be prosthetic and homelike: to emphasize individuals' abilities and maximize independence.

There is provision for twenty-eight permanent residents, with two beds reserved for respite clients. An adult day program was also included, for a maximum of ten participants per day. The original hope was to involve males and females in nearly equal numbers; however, this has not been feasible. The residential population has generally included four to six men (overall, 20 percent of the admissions).

The original residents came from a wide radius, up to two hundred miles away. In some cases, individuals were able to move closer to family or friends, but generally those who came from considerable distances did so because specialized dementia services were not available elsewhere. While small in number, the cross section of clients and the variety of dementia cases have been remarkable. (The clear exception would be in terms of significant ethnic diversity, not characteristic of rural Maine.)

The design includes several separate activity areas and a walking path indoors. Outdoors, there is a specially designed garden. A grassy yard extends around the facility, varying from open lawn, or meadow, to copses of trees—enough to give the impression of being in the woods, which in fact surround the property. (For specific information about the physical design of the facility, see the A.C.C.'s profile in Cohen and Day, *Contemporary Environments for People with Dementia.*)

With the exceptions of locked outer doors and a fairly unobtrusive six-foot fence surrounding the property, the environment, both inside and out, is intended to be as restraint-free as possible: to combine safety and security with a sense of personal freedom. The number of residents receiving any sort of chemical restraint—usually a mild antidepressant or anxiolitic—has generally been small.

The A.C.C. was licensed by the State of Maine as a Special Needs Boarding Home. Individuals served were to be in the early to middle stages of their disease process—often the most challenging in terms of psychosocial needs and behavioral challenges. The actual level, or stage, of those served, though, has always been difficult to quantify. Of the initial resident population, for example, a third were admitted from intermediate-care facilities. Although state criteria for admission to nursing homes are becoming increasingly restrictive, many of our residents over the years would have been placed in intermediate-care facilities if the A.C.C. had not been available.

The original plan was to build an additional long-term care unit to provide a continuum of care on-site. That plan has not yet come to fruition. Therefore, as most dementias are progressive, discharge to another level of care has been inevitable. Some of our more stable individuals have been in their nineties and have presented no symptoms other than "malignant forgetfulness." Persons with dementia, though, are prone to the same age-related health challenges as their peers; most individuals' health problems are not related to dementia.

Admission and discharge criteria hinge on physical considerations.

Basically, individuals have to be reasonably independent with transfer-ring and ambulation to be admitted to A.C.C. They must be willing and able to perform at least some personal care activities with minimal assistance. Eating is a prime example: hand-over-hand cuing during a meal is one thing; actually feeding someone is another. The average length of residence has been two and a half years. A few individuals, suffering drastic physical decline after admission, have been dis-charged after only brief periods; others have remained with us for up to five years.

We do not have hospital beds; there are no bed rails. Our walls lack continuous handrails. By law, we cannot use physical restraints. Often, issues of resident safety become matters for family and staff judgment. For example, with the myoclonic spasms that often develop with de-mentia, individuals become more likely to fall.

Continence is a major issue. Most of those who participate in our programs require at least reminders to maintain continence: either to "think to go" or to remember where the bathrooms are. The majority of residents are on an every-two-hours toileting regimen. Many indi-viduals suffer an increase in "accidents," and even true incontinence, as in bed at night, upon admission. Some never regain their previous levels of independence. Most, however, achieve relative stability. If an individual's physiological incontinence increases—first of urine, then of bowel; first in bed at night, then wholly unawares during the day—then the need for 24-hour nursing care approaches. This is rarely with-out profound deterioration in other bodily systems and cognitive abil-ities.

Often, but by no means always, the bulk of an individual's behav-ioral challenges have subsided by this point. As dementia-specific units are mushrooming throughout Maine (as elsewhere), on discharge the individual has often been able to move to a nursing home closer to home, family, and friends. Nevertheless the transition to a dementia-appropriate nursing facility is often more traumatic for the family (and our staff) than for the individual with dementia.

The Alzheimer's Care Center is part of Kennebec Long Term Care, which also includes two 120-bed intermediate-care facilities. Kennebec Long Term Care is, in turn, a subsidiary of Kennebec Health System, a progressive, comprehensive health-care corporation. The A.C.C. re-ceives various types of administrative support from both companies.

The A.C.C. program has received grants from the Brookdale Foundation and the Robert Wood Johnson Foundation. The adult day program has been a member of Partners in Caregiving, also funded by the Robert Wood Johnson Foundation. The respite service has benefited from federal Health Resources and Services Administration (HRSA) grants.

The Staff

The staff members at the A.C.C. are a uniquely varied bunch. Originally, some came from health care, some from manufacturing, some from homemaking. Ages ranged from twenty to sixty. All shared an interest in working with Alzheimer disease and related dementias. Much of the original staff is still in place.

Logistically, 24-hour staffing follows fairly traditional nursing shifts (7:00 A.M. to 3:00 P.M., 3:00 P.M. to 11:00 P.M., 11:00 P.M. to 7:00 A.M.), with some staggered shifts (6:00 A.M. to 2:00 P.M., 2:00 P.M. to 10:00 P.M., midnight to 8:00 A.M.). There are a charge person (generally a licensed practical nurse) and four aides during the day and evening, and a charge person (a medication technician) and two aides at night.

The support staff includes an administrator and a half-time social worker. (The other half of the social worker's time is spent with the Geriatric Evaluation Unit.) There is a housekeeper between the hours of 7:00 A.M. and 3:30 P.M. A half-time secretary keeps everyone more or less coordinated and provides large quantities of one-to-one time with residents, pets, families, visitors, and others.

There is a forty-hour-a-week activities director position.

Meals are prepared at a nearby, but off-site, hospital kitchen. There is a dietary aide assigned to each meal.

The staff and residents alike depend on a corps of volunteers. The volunteers help out in many ways, from conducting groups, to chaperoning walks, to working with individuals on a one-to-one basis. Individual volunteers provide an average of forty hours of service per week.

Certain aspects of the staff seem to stand out. They tend to be industrious, conscientious workers and not to be working for large financial gain. They are rather autonomous by nature: they work well as team members but can also make appropriate minute-to-minute decisions, and they often love doing so. They are certainly compassionate, and they care deeply for the special individuals whom they assist through the day and night. They take their work seriously and they love a good laugh—in fact, a tendency to laugh too loudly is a common trait. Above all, though, they love a challenge. They enjoy their work precisely because no two days are exactly the same or predictable. They tend to be very inquisitive: searching for new and different approaches or strategies and anxious to try them on for size. They like to analyze what they've done and to try to improve it for the next time. Overall, they love to think, to learn, and to share what they've learned.

The Adult Day Program

Adult day care has been a crucial program of the A.C.C. Participants receive a full range of services. Within the limits of their own preference and choice, they become integrated into the overall program on arrival. Truly, they seem to become one of the family when they walk through the door.

Some participants function at higher levels and enjoy a "helping" role; many perceive their participation to be volunteering. Their involvement sometimes adds a special spark to groups. It also adds frequent challenges in terms of programing for mixed levels of ability. Although adult day program participants must fit the general guidelines for admission, some have been more physically frail than the residents.

Roughly one-third of all adult day program participants have been male. One-quarter of the participants have been subsequently admitted to the A.C.C., with an equal number admitted directly to intermediate or skilled nursing facilities. Roughly half have left the program for other reasons.

The role of the adult day program in helping family members and other home caregivers adapt to and cope with a progressive disease has naturally been enormous. Day respite care has often been the first—and sometimes hardest—step in seeking and accepting outside help. A biweekly support group has continued to be active and significant for those involved.

Respite

Two beds, each in a private room, are reserved for overnight respite. Respite services, offered for one to six weeks, have generally been well utilized, albeit with a decreased demand in the winter.

Those in respite, like adult day program participants, receive a full range of residential services. Every effort is made to meet special needs, to make each individual's stay as normal, as natural-feeling, as possible, and to include the person as much as possible in the overall program.

• About This Book •

When the A.C.C. opened, there was relatively little literature dealing with activity for those with Alzheimer disease and related dementias. There was even less that was practical and applicable to our own situation. Nancy Mace's writings, *The 36-Hour Day* and *Dementia Care*, provided a sound and abiding foundation. Jitka Zgola's pivotal *Doing Things* and Sally Freeman's *Activities and Approaches for Alzheimer's* were both helpful. Zgola's discussion of Alzheimer disease, its characteristics, and general implications for programing remains especially useful.

But no single text, or combination of texts, met all of our needs. Most work in print reflected experiences from adult day programs or those of individual consultants. Most ideas and approaches aside from those cited had not grown beyond the traditional "twin pillars" of the crafts approach and infantilization or, worse, what could be termed "cute-izing" (in which activities at, say, a cognitive age equivalent to the third grade look, feel, and sound like the third grade). Neither dementia nor the aging process is cute.

"There's no book to go by" was a recurring refrain. We continued to learn the most from our residents and adult day program participants: through trial and error, step by learned step. We realized that we were in the process of creating our own body of practical knowledge, and we decided to put it into the form of a manual that could be readily used by caregivers in home-based settings and in facilities for day care, long-term care, and acute care. The intent was to compile, organize, and test specific ideas and techniques that could be easily understood and applied.

This manual is not a cookbook. It is intended to provide ideas, not recipes. Nor is it activity therapy "by the numbers." With any dementia, no two situations, no two victims, caregivers, client groups, staffs, or days will be exactly alike. Dementia is a disease of the brain, so we must use ours. If easy means not thinking, then there are no "easy" approaches to dementia care.

This is, above all, an effort to share what we have found to be helpful in our specific situation, and what we have found less than successful: what tends to work for us, and what has backfired. The general principles contained herein reflect the particular philosophies developed by the A.C.C. staff. They reflect what we have taught and what we continue to utilize on a daily basis. These are the ways in which we keep our folks engaged in the world around them—the world that we help them create, minute by minute, hour by hour, and day by day. These are the tasks and interventions that we use when we have calmly planned a specific group program, and what we grab on the spur of the moment, at 2:00 P.M. or 2:00 A.M.

Much of this material developed spontaneously in group work or on a one-to-one basis. All of it has been honed through direct use. It is hoped that every idea offered here will trigger another for the reader, like ripples spreading out from a pebble tossed into a clear pond. A worthwhile idea should spawn others.

It is essential to be open to new ideas; that's one definition of creativity. Innovation is not so much coming up with unique ideas that nobody else has dreamed of as it is adapting ideas to the needs of each special program and its individuals. It's keeping our eyes, ears, and other senses open. Some of the most innovative ideas are as old as the hills, but with different adaptations. There may be little new under the sun, but with dementia, there are endless new wrinkles.

One occasionally meets a peculiar sort of chauvinism in health care, a "Don't bug us, we're the best," sort of mind-set. Signs include a smug roll of the eyes: "No way. We tried that once and it didn't work," or "Sounds great, but it'd never work with our people," or "What we're doing is already better than that!" Sometimes the longer one works with dementia, the harder it is to stay open to new ideas. However, it's no less important than a physician staying abreast of new medications and procedures, or a parent's adjusting to the changing needs of a growing child. When new ideas have become threatening rather than thrilling, then it is all the more imperative to explore them: "Nothing ventured, nothing gained."

Each caregiver is unique. As caregivers, we each use what could be termed a bag of tricks: our own collection of techniques, approaches, sayings, gestures, facial expressions, and so on. However, we all share certain approaches, as well.

Every facility is unique, and every program is site-specific. But there are similarities, common ground. What does not work today may work tomorrow; what works today may fail tomorrow but might work next Tuesday. What works in Florida should be worth a try in Minnesota.

Little can be done to alter the course of Alzheimer disease or other dementias. However, much can be done to maximize the quality of life of people with dementia. Different treatments have value, depending on the unique situation of each individual. A variety of interventions—an integration that rarely stays static for long—is usually essential. At the moment, however, behavior management, especially constructive, individually appropriate activity, seems to be the most effective approach.

It may be helpful, for a moment, to think of a person as a house. Everyone spends a lifetime decorating and furnishing a unique personal house, the interior reflecting who and what he or she has become. In taking glimpses through the windows, we see the individual. Dementia is a process that draws the curtains in some windows and boards up others. The interior of the house, though, changes little; it may never change much. Our task is to help keep a few windows open, to let the light shine in, at least occasionally. The individual still feels vital on those occasions.

The dark side of dementia can be very dark. The bright side, however, can be brilliant.

Keeping Busy

∴ 1 ∴

Key Ideas

One occupational hazard of working with persons who have dementia is the hope for a "magic wand," a quick, convenient cure for the disease. The question usually sounds like, "Did you hear about that new pill they have? It was on the news last night, or maybe it was in the paper."

The bad news is that at this point there is no panacea. Effective treatments tend to be behavioral, not pharmaceutical. They are time-consuming and inexact; they require constant creativity, inexhaustible patience, vigilance, and energy.

The good news is that what works, usually works. No two humans are alike, and no two will be alike with a dementia. Still, the basics tend to work; there is a "book" to go by. The basics pertain, with appropriate adaptations, throughout the course of the disease. The trick is not so much the book as the style of reading.

• The Basics •

Activity

Activity is a difficult word. Its meaning is not precise. In long-term care, the notions that *activity* usually connotes are too often outmoded. In relation to dementia, those connotations may be irrelevant.

Activity for an individual with dementia should be defined as "everything a person does." Activities include toileting as well as enjoying an old joke, eating as well as watching *I Love Lucy,* putting on a jacket as well as taking a hike. The basic techniques and approaches are identical.

Above all, activity is the responsibility of everyone involved in an individual's care. It cannot be what "someone else" does; it cannot be secondary to anyone's "real" work. Effective care for persons with dementia depends on teamwork.

Structured activities that work with folks who have dementia share two sets of characteristics: they are familiar and they allow people to feel successful.

A task should be "nothing new." It should be something the person has overlearned (performed so many times that it is more or less automatic, or second nature). It should be a "habitual skill," an "automatic program" (Zgola, 1987). Common examples are raking the lawn, sweeping the floor, chopping vegetables, wiping tables, drying dishes, folding washcloths, winding wire.

Music, sayings, or discussion topics should be what the person knew before the dementia set in. Folks are unlikely to newly learn to use a walker or a call-bell. If a person never wore turtlenecks, now is not the time to start. Replacing shoelaces with Velcro may be a godsend to the caregiver, but bewildering to the person with dementia.

Tasks well rehearsed as an avocation rather than a vocation may be more successful. The important thing may be not what an individual has overlearned but what he or she enjoyed overlearning. Washing dishes is not a comforting task to some; not all homeowners love mowing the lawn. Many enthusiastic cooks are thrilled to retire from the kitchen. A career waitress might not enjoy wiping down the tables before or after lunch. A stitching card may be the last thing a shoe-stitcher of fifty years would welcome (especially if the card looks infantile to start with).

Historical interests can be tricky, however. The former radio repair person, presented with a dysfunctional old radio, may well perceive his or her lost capabilities and send the offending appliance hurtling past the well-meaning caregiver's left ear. The career secretary is unlikely to be satisfied with her or his present typing.

The strongest attraction for folks with dementia is to succeed, to have a chance to shine. "Aha! I can do that!" is more appealing than, "Oh, I used to do that."

Any task that appears helpful will likely feel successful. No phrase is more motivating than "I need your help." As one gentleman commented, "There's no limit to what I'll do—if I can do it!"

A task, naturally, should be of an appropriate cognitive level. It may challenge, but it should not frustrate. If an individual attempts a task that is too demanding, he or she will likely show signs of rising frustration. Because most folks tend to gravitate toward tasks appropriate to both their abilities and their interests, most are more than happy to be assisted in shifting to another, more doable, task. (Since "Good try" implies failure, the caregiver may simply say, "Thank you," or "O.K., great," or "You know, I forgot about this: could you help me do this first?")

Each individual is different, and today will not be precisely like yesterday or last Friday. Most folks, however, will need to be engaged in some activity, or occupied, at least once every half hour. Naturally there are individuals who will sit placidly, hands folded neatly in their laps, almost for hours at a time. There are others who require constant supervision.

Work

Webster's dictionary defines *work* as "physical or mental effort directed toward a goal; the activity that serves as one's . . . occupation." The concept of continuing to work is crucial in maintaining "balance" with dementia.

The most valuable dementia activity is work that is tied to the life of the home (whether institution or private home). The key is making work: thinking in terms of "long cuts" rather than the shortcuts that our normal routines demand. Keeping someone calm and busy is often a near-constant process of distraction: diverting an individual's focus from a source of anxiety, redirecting a problem behavior. Very often, the most important question a caregiver can ask, whether at home or in a group setting, is, "What can a resident/loved one do to help me with what I'm doing now?"

We cringe at the term *busywork:* work arranged, or created, for the sake of being busy. That is, however, the key to keeping folks with a dementia occupied. Busywork is demeaning only if it feels like busywork. The promise of success that a task offers usually outweighs the actual goals—or lack of them.

Achievement, being useful, is the most motivating thing of all: "Aha,

I can do this!" generally overrides any other concern, including whether a given task might be "men's" or "women's" work. If a task engages an individual—if it "works"—then it is purposeful.

Behavior Management

It has been said that most problem behaviors with dementia are the result of poor behavior management. Management for a person with dementia begins with the environment. It is useful to make a distinction between personal and external environments. If someone is in pain, sleep deprivation, or urgent need of a bowel movement, then such a personal environment is the primary concern. Factors such as the weather, phase of the moon, barometric pressure, and time of day are relevant, too. If nothing is amiss in the personal sphere, then the concern shifts to the external setting.

In a prosthetic, dementia-appropriate environment, behavior management generally means keeping the individual occupied. This, in turn, means being busy enough without being too busy, without becoming overly tired. There should be a constant pattern of "on/off," stress/release, busyness/relaxation. The relaxed periods may be shorter than the active ("Quiet Hour" at the A.C.C. is rarely sixty minutes long). Successive group programs may last as long as an hour; the rest between them may well last less than fifteen minutes.

A major standard for programing recreation in the long-term care field deals with the quality and availability of appropriate independent activity. Unfortunately, the concept of independent activity is largely irrelevant, even counterproductive, with dementia. Generally, if individuals with dementia are left alone to independent pursuits, they will "wind up"—grow increasingly nervous, agitated, angry, terrified. Left untreated, these symptoms can result in a catastrophic reaction, often a confrontation between two "wound-up" people. Dementia may not be contagious, but anxiety definitely is. Anxiety can be thought of as simply being out of balance: the person has lost equilibrium. The environment no longer makes sense; everything is out of whack. An old psychological term for this is "cognitive dissonance." The most common manifestation of being out of balance is the urge to "go home."

It is essential to be proactive. Proacting simply means thinking ahead, anticipating, rather than waiting to react. Proacting is intervening before there is a problem, before the smoke becomes a flame. It is the foundation of a prosthetic environment. A minute of proaction is worth an hour of reaction. The observation, "It's calm now," requires the question, "What will we be doing in twenty minutes?"

Control

Control is a central issue in everyone's life. It underlies most achievement, most of the hassles between parent and teenager, and most marital friction. "Control refers to our need to make an impact on our environment, that is, to move things in the direction of our own choosing" (Zgola, 1987, p. 28).

For all of us, lack of control in our lives is always frustrating, even infuriating. Dementias can strip individuals of their ability to control their world. Small choices, then, become important. The more choice they can exercise, the more control they perceive. And the more control they perceive, the greater sense of independence and self-esteem they enjoy.

Decision making can be very frustrating for individuals with dementia. The only thing more infuriating is not being given a choice. The classic reply, "Oh, I don't care, dear: You decide," is often a plea to be allowed to choose. Some individuals truly do not care to make a choice in a given situation. Usually, though, it is amazing how immediate and clear a decision is, if the person is offered the choice a second time.

Most folks can exercise some degree of choice regardless of dementia and regardless of the stage of the disease. There is, however, a hierarchy of ability to choose that depends on the individual and his or her cognitive condition. All rules regarding communication and behavior still apply. A person who is already agitated or has a headache is not likely to make a choice. If the setting is rushed, or noisy, or busy, then one may be less likely to choose anything (other than to depart).

Many occasions for offering choices occur naturally throughout the day. The caregiver's decision to ask the questions depends on the individual's overall cognitive ability, as well as ability at the moment. Requests to the person to make choices will rarely be frustrating if the person does not feel overwhelmed or badgered. It is seldom wise to offer a choice—in the same manner, anyway—more than twice.

What color of clothing to wear may represent the first choice of the day. We'll assume that Christina wants a sweater, today or in general, and that she will need some assistance with putting it on. We should also assume that the caregiver has established and maintained an effective rapport with her. (If not, the caregiver should no longer be attempting to accomplish the task of helping Christina to dress herself.) The following questions range from open choice to closed choice.

- "Christina, which of your sweaters would you like to wear this morning?" (Depending on her verbal abilities, Christina could at any step be invited to point to the sweater of her choice.)

- "Christina, here are your sweaters [in the closet]. Which one would you like to wear this morning?" The caregiver will need to take the sweaters out of the closet and present them. As a rule, the maximum number of items among which folks with dementia can choose is three. Choosing among more than three is almost always confusing, no matter how highly functioning the individual may be.

- Let's assume that a choice between two is most appropriate for Christina. "Christina, which sweater would you like to wear this morning? This one, blue, or this one, red?"

- "Christina? I know you like to wear a sweater in the morning. Do you like red?" or "Do you like this sweater?" A yes/no decision ("Do you want this?") is still a choice.

Another example of a hierarchy of questions may be found in a "picnic" situation.

Three types of sandwiches are arranged on separate trays. The sandwiches are on dark bread or white bread and are halved. Helpers stand behind the table or with the client to assist (and to handle the food). Individuals' choices to be "waited on" at their table are usually respected; this does not eliminate their opportunity to choose. Eye contact, the level and cadence of the voice, etc., and other signals are important, but let's focus on the decision-making.

- "Hello, Amos. We have sandwiches. We have tuna, peanut butter and jelly, and egg salad. Would you like one, or would you like a combination?"

- "Hello, Gil. We have sandwiches. Do you like tuna or peanut butter and jelly?" If Gil was able to choose between the two items, then the item he preferred can be paired with the third item. So, if he chose tuna, the next choice could be tuna or egg. The assumption is that the individual has made an appropriate choice: that, in this case, Gil does not care for peanut butter.

Through the middle stages of dementia, most individuals can readily choose between two items. The choice of dark bread or white is often easier than the type of sandwich: to some, it is a more visual choice; to others, a more definite preference. This, then, adds more choice—and more achievement—to the proceedings

- "Hello, Lili. We have sandwiches. Do you like tuna?" If she shows a dislike for tuna, the next choice could be offered. If all choices are turned down, another message may be clear: Lili may not be hungry, may not like sandwiches, or may be in no mood to eat to begin with! She is still expressing a decision.

The individual who "parrots" a choice—repeating the last item he or she heard—is nonetheless making a decision and will still feel successful.

Visual cues can be strengthened in many ways. Open-face sandwiches ("displayed") may be more meaningful than the words *egg salad*. Signs denoting the choices are helpful to some (and may be picked up in lieu of a sandwich). Individuals can often point to condiments—mustard, mayonnaise, ketchup, etc.—more easily than verbally expressing a preference.

Opportunities for choice should be woven into structured activities during the day. The typical coffee/snacks/juice cart can offer choice as well as "a little something" to ensure nutrition and hydration. A typical hierarchy of choice might be as follows:

- "What would you like to drink?" (bearing in mind that such an open-ended question invites responses ranging from water to root beer to Scotch and soda).
- "Would you like coffee or juice?"
- "Would you like something hot or something cold?" (If coffee, then, "With milk? sugar?" If juice, then, "Orange or apple?")
- "Which do you want?" (showing the individual two visual choices).

- "Would you like some juice?" (Sometimes, at this point, a choice between two alternatives can still be made, either verbally or visually.)
- "Do you want this?" ("Thirsty?")
- A single choice can be offered with appropriate gestures and facial expressions.

A quick and easy "choice" activity can be to fill three pitchers with a colorless soft drink (such as ginger ale) or water. Then, add a little food coloring to two (or all) of the pitchers. It can be astonishing to watch folks' interest in and deliberations among the colored liquids. Presweetened powdered beverages can be used to the same end, but unsweetened powders offer the benefit of needing to have sugar added: there is usually at least one person who will gladly open sugar packets to provide sweetening.

• General Approaches •

The following is a list of dos and don'ts for interacting with an individual with dementia, gleaned from our experience at the A.C.C. Some are old; some are not. Some are common sense; some are not. It is rare that a day goes by without our using these principles at least twice.

- Show respect; treat me as an adult.
  Don't "baby" me.
- Smile!
  Don't show me your stress.
- Enable me.
  Don't "do for me."
- Know the individual.
  Don't assume that I'm like anyone else.
- Expect the unexpected.
  Don't assume anything.
- Stay calm; keep "our" cool.
  Don't panic.
- Let me take my own sweet time.
  Don't rush me—or else!
- Move slowly; don't rush.
  Don't scare me; there's no fire.

- Let me follow my own routine.
  Don't inflict your schedule on me!
- Ensure my success.
  Don't give me a task that I may not be able to accomplish.
- Be proactive (anticipate).
  Don't wait to react.
- Create work.
  Don't think in terms of short cuts.
- Create chances for choice.
  Don't forget all of the above.
- If you want to get my attention or stop me from doing
    something, call my name.
  Don't say "No!"
- Say, "Please."
  Don't order me around.
- Change the subject.
  Don't argue.
- Stoop to my eye level.
  Don't make me look up your nose.
- Tickle my sense of humor.
  Don't be afraid to be silly
- Remember: "My dementia made me do it."
  Don't scold me.
- Remember: I have a dementia.
  Don't take it personally!

• Orientation to Time and Place •

Staff members are the clocks and calendars for folks with dementia. Incidental repetition of the time of day, day of the week, date, month, season, and so on is helpful throughout the day. "Let's see. Today is Friday, so we might be having fish for lunch," or "Isn't this a perfect summer morning?" is not likely to trigger anxiety. Reality orientation is often the cornerstone of an effective discussion or "cognitive stimulation" group. Although folks with dementia generally want to know the basic time orientation, they do not want to be contradicted. "Old-fashioned" reality orientation (see Appendix A) never taught anyone to argue with a client.

A reality-orientation board displays basic facts in a simple, uncluttered, noninfantile style. Black lettering on a white background continues to be the color combination participants choose as being easiest to read. Such display boards, or kiosks, are readily available commercially or can be easily made. A.C.C. uses the less-than-innovative format of a corkboard and push-pins, with a combination of store-bought and hand-made cards or posters. Most commercially available boards are geared toward the elementary school classroom and tend to be both childish and "busy" (cluttered with colors, abstract designs, cartoon figures, etc.).

The various calendars plainly visible near the checkout at your local market (to help "normal" individuals remember this information and avoid the mortification of having to ask) are useful, though the graphic arrangement may not make sense to an older viewer.

October
W E D N E S D A Y
15th

This kind of information is best offered incidentally, "take it or leave it," to the viewers. The process (as with traditional reality orientation) should be one of gentle reminding, not teaching or persuasion or memorization. The group leader may suggest that the information is there to help him or her, which may not be far from the truth.

Folks will often read reality-orientation boards independently throughout the day (and each time may seem like the first time). I have never seen or heard anyone react badly to these basic facts. Some individuals may express surprise at the day or month, but most are usually glad to know the truth.

The use of information regarding place, though, can be problematical. For example, we no longer mention our city, Gardiner, on our board. When used in the past, it occasionally reminded someone that he or she had to "get home": "This is Gardiner? Well, I live in Podunk, and my people will be worried. I have to get going!"

Folks with dementia feel either at home or not at home, minute to minute, hour to hour. In our situation, including the state (Maine) often triggers feelings of pleasure and pride, although on occasion—with individuals from another state—it has provoked some anxiety.

A typical arrangement of information might be:

It's Autumn

(The leaves haven't fallen.)

Today is **Monday.** It's wash day!

October Xth 199x

We're in the state of **Maine!**

Oral repetition of each item seems to help folks register the information. This can be achieved simply. For example: "Yesterday was Sunday, so of course today is . . ." Or, pointing at the day, "Somebody please help me remember what day it is." An adapted pep cheer could be useful: "Give me an M, give me an O, give me an N, [etc.]."

Each of these items creates possibilities for discussions. For example, each day has certain traditional associations. Some people are quick to offer ideas and recollections about the old-fashioned Monday "wash day." This is especially true if the group leader suggests that no one present could be old enough to remember using a washboard (or scrub board). A suggestion that rarely fails to get a rise out of the group is that the men would traditionally do the Monday laundry and give the women a well-deserved day off.

Other supports, or "anchors," for recalling the days of the week include special foods: "Monday is Italian sandwich day"; "If we're having doughnuts, then it must be Wednesday"; "Friday is fish day"; "It's Saturday: we're having beans for supper!"

A list of seasonal activities, retaining a core of items day after day, provides opportunity for both information and reminiscing. For example: "As we've been saying [perhaps mentioning who contributed what items during a previous session or sessions], autumn is a busy time. In autumn, people rake leaves, wash windows, pick apples, clean up the garden, finish the canning." Someone might add, "And pick the tomatoes"; someone else, "Go to school"; and so on.

• Scheduling •

The most important thing about scheduling a program for persons with dementia is the routine, not the schedule per se. The actual time of an event is not important; the sequence of events is. The hallmark of an activity schedule that is appropriate for a person with dementia is consistency: daily, weekly, and monthly. What might be mind-numbing redundancy to a caregiver may well be independence-sustaining predictability to the person with dementia.

No one staff member, volunteer, or family member can effectively conduct a specific activity at the same time, in the same way, every day—at least, not for long. That is a sure formula for becoming at best stale and at worst burned out. The problem with burnout is that by the time we (or our co-workers) realize that we've been "singed," it's too late to avoid it.

Some activities by their nature should be scheduled with consistency and frequency. Exercise routines, for example, could actually be dangerous if conducted only once or twice a week. In general, while weekly might be good with some programs, daily is probably better. Some folks will learn a certain song, sung by a specific volunteer, every Tuesday afternoon. More folks will learn it, though, and will learn it faster, if it's sung three times a week, and more yet if it's sung daily. As with everyone else, the more they learn, the more they use their memory, the more slowly they will lose it. This is not to say that there can't be variety; we all need that! Special events are always special, and even more so if we can anticipate them. It is to say, though, that any schedule for persons with dementia should contain routine and predictability in its daily and weekly structure.

A basic consideration in programing for dementia is simply what is "normal." Most people think better after exercising, so exercise should precede a discussion group. We all tend to be mentally sharpest in the late morning, so memory games probably should be conducted then. The world loves a midmorning break—coffee, juice, etc.—and a late-afternoon "pick-me-up" snack. Programing should also anticipate the increased fatigue of late afternoon, and especially the potentially catastrophic effect of the 3:00 P.M. shift change in health care facilities.

Effective activity programing for dementia often depends, too, on parallel programing. This is true in both specialized units and mixed populations, day care or residential. No one program or modality will occupy everyone, ever. A "core" group will involve most individuals, but a second, smaller group will often be required as well. This does not so much create a choice as offer more individual-appropriate alternatives. Once a group activity is under way, the most important questions become "Who *isn't* involved?" and "Do they need to be occupied?"

Individual or one-to-one activity will ensure that everyone is effectively occupied. If two individuals are disturbed by the commotion of a given entertainment, they might be willing instead to help prepare a snack for later. Another individual might prefer to have a cup of coffee with a staff member—or simply to sit by herself—in a quiet spot. Someone else might be taking a nap, another quite happily strolling indoors or out in the garden. Common examples of parallel programing include dayroom sessions, for those unable to be involved in a centralized ("rec room") program, and bedside or in-room activity as needed.

Core programs can include very traditional (though more or less specially adapted) offerings such as group exercise, adapted sports and games, musical entertainments, slide programs, films, discussions, parties, and so on. Most such activities can be adapted to both small group and one-to-one situations.

The different groups may well last for varying lengths of time, and some individuals may shift from one to another and back again. It is important to note that neither large nor small groups are generally conducted back-to-back; there is usually a rest period in between.

A helpful guideline in planning dementia-appropriate activity is the "fifteen-minute model." Caregivers sometimes say, discouraged, "I can't find anything that will occupy him for more than fifteen minutes at a time!" A task that does occupy someone for fifteen minutes, however, should be considered successful. Three more tasks, or the same one repeated, would create a well-occupied hour. Of course, each quarter-hour segment might be separated by a walk around, a look out the window, a drink of water, a trip to the bathroom, etc.

The nature of our daily routine often interests visitors to the A.C.C. A frequent reaction has been, "It's so normal. It's like the real world." And so it is, in ways. The basic schedule is shown in Appendix B. It may need minor seasonal adjustments. Our weekend schedule also varies a bit. To some extent this reflects decreased staff and volunteer support as well as a smaller number of adult day program participants.

Our original assumption was that the regular daily activity routine should carry over to Saturday and Sunday as well. However, early efforts to involve residents in the "regular" morning exercise group met with a notable lack of interest on weekends. It rapidly became obvious that our residents wanted—perhaps needed—a morning of rest, come Saturday morning. It became equally obvious, however, that we did need to adhere to the established routine of a midmorning coffee/ snack break!

The rest of the weekend generally follows the weekly routine. On Sundays, the group programs are usually devotional, hymn-singing groups and formal (somewhat specialized) worship services.

• Steps in a Structured Group Activity •

Some basic guidelines for structuring time will pertain, whether the activity to be undertaken is a whirlpool bath or a large-group discussion. Two of the most valuable studies for anyone working with a population with dementia are basic remotivation training and basic lesson planning as used by successful classroom teachers. There is an obvious similarity, in the procedure outlined here, to the steps in the traditional Remotivation Method (see Appendix C). The standard remotivation technique, like all other approaches, often needs adaptation to maximize its success for people with dementia. However, flexibility has always been one of the beauties of this tried-and-true system (and its practitioners).

At first, we were not sure what role group programing would play in our overall program. As our initial admissions arrived individually (never more than two per day), it seemed feasible to base the activity program on individual involvement. However, it soon grew apparent that keeping everyone sufficiently busy, strictly or even primarily with individual activities, was going to be a daunting task indeed.

Happily, we soon realized that group programing could—in fact, did—have a very significant impact. Individuals whom families had described as "loners" or "anxious in social settings" did surprisingly well and even thrived in groups. Many individuals grew to be more secure within a social group than they were on their own. A clear sense of security, of "safety in numbers," became apparent: Sally Freeman's useful concept of "group-ness" (Freeman, 1987).

An obvious advantage of group activity as opposed to individual activity is that groups can allow a fairly low ratio of staff to residents. An effective group leader can involve twenty or more individuals for as long as an hour. Of course, the group has to be seen as a collection of individuals.

The following is by way of a recipe for success with a dementia-appropriate event.

Preparation

Preparation is at least 80 percent of success and includes planning, scheduling, assembling materials, and set up. Preparation for dementia programming must be minimized. In teaching and in Therapeutic Activity Work, a fifty-fifty trade-off may sometimes be required: an hour's preparation for an hour's actual programming. The intensity of a dementia schedule, however, makes even a two-to-one ratio (half an hour's prep to an hour's programming) impractical. The fact that material and ideas can be re-cycled frequently is an enormous ally. This drastically reduces *Planning* tasks such as telephone time, volunteer coordinating, research, and materials acquisition.

Scheduling determines the best time for this activity in light of what's best for the individual, in relation to the rest of the day's goings-on, the weather, etc.

Materials needed will include information, lists of questions, sayings and so on, music, pictures, posters, decorations and other audio-visual aides, manipulative/hands-on objects or other props.

Set-up includes the arrangement of materials, equipment, furniture, lighting, ventilation, controlling background noise, etc. The best arrangements for a group involve curved lines: a circle, semicircle, or horseshoe. Among other things, this makes it easier for the group leader and others to move, affords maximal eye contact, assists the hearing-impaired, and lets participants pass items from one person to the next.

An especially effective setup consists of tables (such as the standard folding variety) arranged in a horseshoe or three-sided shape. Participants, whether in chairs, in wheelchairs, or standing, gather around the outside of the tables, facing in, while the leader works on the inside. This facilitates using discussion objects, manipulatives or pictures (perhaps laminated or in plastic page protectors).

Success also depends on *anticipating individual needs*. Residents with sensory challenges may need to be close to the group leader; those who will likely leave after ten minutes should be able to do so with minimal commotion; the man who enjoys the role of doorperson should be at his "station"; the woman who is sensitive to drafts should be safely away from the windows.

It is especially important to turn all chairs around to face the program being presented. Few people with dementia ever think to turn a chair around. Most will actually sit through an entire entertainment program, never once turning either the chair or their head to see it. Some will become disinterested (not surprisingly) and depart, even if they would love the goings-on if they saw them.

Referrals (who should be involved, who probably should not) will be an important preparatory decision. In the selection process it is useful to think in terms of "spark plugs." These are the most volatile, the most likely to create a confrontation, to become agitated, to suddenly turn panic-stricken or distraught if not occupied. Some individuals will always be prone to problems if not almost constantly involved; others will vary from day to day.

In any group of individuals, some will need more attention than others. The key is to involve individuals proactively, before they escalate from anxiety to agitation. Once they become "wound up," group involvement is often not feasible. There are those, as well, for whom group involvement is rarely—perhaps never—feasible. There are some whose maximal group involvement is passive, as during a musical entertainment, with one-to-one support, and then for no more than fifteen minutes.

As a rule, any organized activity should include one or more "spark plugs." If not involved in a core group activity, they should be otherwise occupied. Assume, for example, that a van outing is planned, for which none of the "spark plugs" is felt to be appropriate. Alma is just getting over the flu and would become too exhausted, Dominic might not be able to handle the necessary walking (and refuses to use a wheelchair), Rita would almost certainly be overstimulated, Walt hates riding to begin with, and Carlotta was up all night and just got to sleep. Assume, also, that canceling the outing is not a viable option and that those who are going will have a wonderful time. It would obviously be vital to arrange for the others to have something else to do in the meantime. It's not a matter of spoiling people, it's not rewarding problem behaviors; it's preventing them to begin with.

Many people, with or without dementia, have a habit of busyness, and no amount of activity satisfies them. The busier some individuals are, the more they will complain of boredom. These do not, however, tend to be the explosive, "spark plug" types. Most individuals do not grow more demanding with appropriate activity intervention; it is simply what they need to stay calm.

Finally, preparation must include *announcing*—informing staff members of what's coming up and informing residents who can recall independently that the event will be starting at such-and-such a time (say, two minutes or half an hour in advance).

Gathering the Group

Motivation to join a group activity can be approached in many ways, all of which may be needed in a particular instance. It includes informing individuals that the event is about to start; reminding the staff that the time is nigh; asking for one person's help; reminding another of the special contribution he or she had promised to make; reassuring another that he or she is wanted and/or needed; accepting another's decision to remain "at rest"—and asking again in two minutes.

It is always important to recall, however wonderful the specific program might be or however perfectly suited it might be to a given individual, that the most motivating thing tomorrow will often be our acceptance of "No, I'd rather not . . .," today.

For *transportation* (guiding/assisting folks as needed to the area of the event), a team of two works best: one (at least) gathering participants and one "anchor" to stay with those already assembled, greet newcomers, and arrange strategic seating. For one leader to gather an entire group of ambulatory individuals—to gather an appropriate number of "spark plugs" and others—is often like filling a bucket with a gaping hole in the bottom.

Greeting/Beginning

The greeting is the "hook"; it grabs everyone's attention. This step could be called "Sing and Smile."

It is helpful to think of Step 1 of the basic remotivation technique. It is essential to create a "climate of acceptance": a feeling of comfort, of social security, the promise of achievement and/or enjoyment for each individual.

Depending on the size of the group, it may be possible to address each individual at the outset. (One of our staff members uses a unique talent in beginning each group by going around the circle or room and creating a two-line rhyme about each individual.) In any event it is usually possible—and important—to establish eye contact, to "trade smiles," with everyone. There will be key group members who are essential to contact; these definitely include the "spark plugs."

It is crucial to get most, if not all, of the group immediately involved. Involvement is attention. The more passive an individual's involvement, the more likely he or she is to be distracted by something other than the event at hand. A simple "Good Morning" or "Hello," repeated several times until a rousing chorus is achieved, can be effective. Clapping often catches on; laughter can also demand attention. A simple poem or saying, known to all, can also work (especially engaging, at times, if the group leader requires "assistance" in recalling each succeeding line). A familiar song can work wonders.

Any similarities between this step and the beginning of a comedian's routine or the television audience "warm-up" before a quiz show is no coincidence.

The Program

1. Introduction/Stimulus

    Once the group's attention is established, the introductory step presents the actual event: what will follow, an overview of "what we're going to be doing."

2. The First Task

    Introduce the first task to be done: the first question, work-task, song, article of clothing to be removed, etc. Often the group leader should give one or more examples.

3. Reinforce the Task Done

    "Great Job! Thank you!"

4. Repeat Steps 2 and 3 as needed

5. Closure (The End)

    Remotivation technique is helpful in the conclusion. Again, a "climate of acceptance" is important. This should include a review and reinforcement of what has transpired, reminders of individual contributions, statements, wisecracks, and so on. It is also important to provide a transition to the next activity period, or sequence. Each activity, however structured or informal, needs to flow from, and into, another.

A Few Guidelines for a Structured Activity

- Have all materials at hand when the program begins.
- Use names as much as possible. It provides reassurance and helps individuals to maintain attentiveness.
- Maintain eye contact (except, at times, during personal care).
- Play dumb sometimes. "Gosh, I wonder . . . " can go a long way. (But don't play dumb during personal care; be competent and inspire a feeling of confidence.)
- Ask universal questions: "How many people here have ever had a dog?" "Who likes apple pie?" "How many here ever went to school?" "How many ever rode in a car?"
- Try to recall individual interests, past achievements, abilities, etc.
- Go with the flow. If a dog strolls into the group, shift the discussion: talk about it, emphasize its name and owner, perhaps sing *Doggie in the Window*.
- Acknowledge all contributions ("Thank you for asking," "Thanks for adding that," etc.).
- Repeat what participants say, as much as possible "in their own words." This not only reinforces the value of an individual's contribution but also serves to amplify and translate, or interpret, if necessary, the statements for the rest of the group.
- To maintain (or regain) control in a group, try speaking more slowly and more deliberately, and with a deeper tone.
- Have more material on hand than you can use (other options to fall back on).
- If all else fails, sing a song!

·: 2 :·

Humor

The goals of the activities program are to create immediate pleasure, restore dignity, provide meaningful tasks, restore roles and
enable friendship. In fact, one could say that the goal of the activity
therapist is to enable his or her clients to laugh.

Nancy L. Mace (1987)

Dementia is nothing to laugh about. However, as one individual with
dementia observed, "If we can't laugh, I guess we can't . . . do much."

Most jokes about dementia are, in fact, crudely insulting, and they
tend to be both ageist and sexist. Smiling at our own failings—regarding memory and otherwise—can be healthy. Being insulted, being
laughed at, is not.

Humor for the caregiver is, above all, an attitude, an approach. It
means not taking ourselves or our pressures too seriously. An A.C.C.
resident commented, "Life is too serious to be serious. You gotta have
a laugh once in a while." Taking the risk of being "silly" is not a habit
that most health care professionals have acquired.

The field of humor as a therapeutic technique continues to blossom,
if not explode, in terms of publications. The knowledge that humor
can be a major factor in good health and recovery is not new: "A merry
heart doeth good like a medicine: but a broken spirit drieth the bones"
(Proverbs 17:22). "Good humor" in medieval medicine applied to a
balance of what were viewed as the four main bodily fluids, or "hu-
mors." In recent years, laughter has been clinically implicated in controlling pain, strengthening the immune system, enhancing memory,

and so on. The mind-body connection is often seen as hinging on humor.

The most basic point to bear in mind is that humor with dementia begins with a smile. It often need go no further. Few interventions are more motivating, more reassuring, more enabling, than a smile. Smiling is one of our earliest learned social skills, and it can be one of the most durable as dementia progresses.

A laugh is simply the next step. Smiling feels good; laughing feels great! It releases tension, dilutes stress, induces relaxation. If I lack short-term recall, a smile or a laugh can quickly change my mood. Humor helps us cope, or at least feel as though we're coping.

However, humor and/or laughter may well be the best cognitive exercise. Laughter has been referred to as "internal stationary jogging" (W. Fry, quoted in Robinson, 1989). As with other cognitive abilities, humor follows certain more or less predictable steps in developing. Fourth-grade humor is different from fifth-grade humor. "Adult" humor is something that we grow into; most children appreciate the Three Stooges more than the Marx brothers. With dementia, humor, like other cognitive skills, follows similar steps in reverse. Folks can appreciate a bad joke or a terrible pun after they have lost the ability to "joke around" verbally; they can enjoy laughing along with a group long after they have lost the ability to actually comprehend the cause of the laughter.

Visual humor is more effective still. It's too bad that pies in the face are so messy, because they almost guarantee mirth. A funny hat or an exaggerated facial expression is worth a hundred words. Jack Benny got more laughs by simply staring than by saying anything. It is important, however, to differentiate between physical humor and what might appear violent. A funny walk or a pratfall might be funny; much of the Three Stooges material can be quite disturbing.

Dementia-appropriate humor is "friendly," positive. It insults no one and nothing. In other words, it is good-natured, "kind and gentle." The TV show *M.A.S.H.* and, in particular, the character of Dr. Pierce provide an example of what dementia humor must *not* be: black, gallows humor. This tough, grim, ironic, "survival" humor may be healthy in a nursing home staff room or a high school teachers' lounge, but not with individuals or groups with dementia.

Humor with dementia should also be broad—the bigger, the better.

Laughter for dementia tends to be booming in nature, a belly-laugh. Exaggeration (hyperbole) is an aid to comprehension. Much "grandfather," or tall-tale, humor is of this nature.

Humor should be familiar. In a family, individuals have certain predictable "lines" that they say. Young children may groan, but they eagerly anticipate hearing Dad say the same old thing at a predictable moment. At the A.C.C., staff members develop such lines, or sayings, as well. Some are specific to each caregiver; some are specific to each resident. That is, we all use the same line to get Sophie to grin, just as everyone would use (or not use) a certain nickname.

The more often a funny line is said, the funnier it will tend to be. Thank goodness, what's funny today will likely be funny tomorrow! The same amusing comment or joke can be used over and over. Here are some of the more frequently heard "lines" around the A.C.C. The more they're used, and the more familiar they were to begin with, the heartier a laugh they tend to get.

- "Gunnar shouldn't have a doughnut; he's too sweet already! If he gets any sweeter, he'll melt in the shower!" (Not to be used referring to a diabetic person!)
- "I've been getting my *mords wixed* all morning."
- "Is everyone here at least sixteen years of age?"
- "How many people here were children at one time?"
- "I come from a large family: I have thirty-four brothers. Mom named us all John. It helps when she wants to call us in for supper."
- Mabel, the 20-foot pet chicken (and related household predicaments).
- "I can't hear you; my glasses are dirty!"
- "I can't hear you; I have a banana in my ear!" (with or without a prop).
- "Wait till you get to be *my* age; I'm a hundred and eighty!" (The more absurd the age exaggeration, the better: a staff member stating her age as a hundred and three is funny; a hundred and sixty is funnier.)
- "You walk [or whatever] like you've been doing it all your life!"
- "Oh, [person entering the room, or group's name]. Thank good-

ness! We just walked to [some distant but well-known city], looking for you!"

* "I'd offer you a cup of tea if I knew you were at least 18!"

Word play is another frequently successful type of humor. Malapropisms ("chief cook and battle wisher") or spoonerisms ("butcher, baker, and candlemake sticker") have a humorous element, and also give folks a chance to "correct" whoever got the mords wixed!

"Good old songs" lend themselves to such mangling. Examples are *My Wild Irish* Nose or *Let Me* Sweet *You* Call *Heart.*

• Jokes •

Smiling, as well as the ability to laugh and appreciate humor, has little or nothing to do with telling, comprehending, or appreciating jokes. Some very funny jokes are told well by individuals with no real sense of humor; other very witty people can never remember a joke to tell! Not all comedians, professional or otherwise, are funny people.

Actual jokes, though, may teach us more about dementia humor than anything else. This is not to say that all caregivers should play comedian all day. But the nature of jokes that "work" suggests what kind of humor is appropriate to dementia.

"Knock, knock" jokes generally do not work with dementia. These are multistep jokes, and they rarely get beyond the second ("Who's there?") or third ("'Sam and Janet' who?") step. However, if just one participant can follow along with the steps of these jokes, then others will get the punchline, usually a pun.

Dementia jokes should, above all, be "as old as the hills." Luckily, the same jokes can be told over and over, day after day; one does not have to find new material every day. And when someone anticipates a punchline or groans in recognition, it's a great moment!

Many old, corny jokes were staples of minstrel shows and vaudeville; many still make the rounds of elementary schools. Some version of "Why did the chicken cross the road?" could probably be found on Sumerian tablets and the walls of the Pharaohs' tombs.

A number of magazines publish appropriate jokes or riddles, ranging from *Highlights for Children* to *Reader's Digest* to the *National Inquirer.* Libraries usually have a variety of joke and riddle books.

Here are some examples of old jokes (in short versions, which can of course be drawn out). While these depend on very limited short-term memory, it is usually helpful to repeat the first line immediately before the punchline.

- Why did the frog cross the road?
  —Because it was tied to the chicken!
- Why did the golfer wear two pairs of pants?
  —In case he got a hole in one!
- How do you get down off a horse?
  —You don't. You get down off a goose!
- Did you hear about the dentist and the carpenter? They got married. It didn't work out, though; they fought tooth and nail!
- What do you do if your pet elephant hurts its toe?
  —Call a toe truck!
- Why did the elephant sit on the marshmallow?
  —He didn't want to fall into the hot chocolate!
- A man bursts into a psychiatrist's office and says, "Doc, Doc, you gotta help me! My wife thinks she's a piano!" The doctor says, "Have no fear: I can cure your wife. Just bring her in for an appointment." "What?" the man yells. "Do you have any idea how much it costs to move a piano these days?"
- Did you hear about the snow tires John bought?
  —They were so cheap they melted!
- How do you make a cow fly?
  —Buy her a plane ticket!
- How do you make a butterfly?
  —Throw it out the window!
- What happens when ducks fly upside-down?
  —They quack up!
- A man bursts into a psychiatrist's office and yells, "Doc, Doc, you gotta help me! I think I'm a dog!" "I can cure you," the doctor says confidently. "You'll never think you're a dog again. Just lie down on my couch." "Oh, no!" the man yells. "I can't; I'm not allowed on the furniture!"

• A Bad Idea: Clowns •

Clowns can be a bad idea. They are very apt to seem "childish" (though this can be less threatening if there are children present). And the outlandish costumes and exaggerated facial make-up can be terrifying—like masks to a three-year-old.

• A Puzzlement •

I once found a book at the local library which had a title like *15,001 Sure-fire Jokes for After-dinner Speakers*. Most of the witticisms in this particular volume were sure-fire duds. No matter how I changed the set-up or the punchline, or dramatized or personalized the stories, I could barely milk a chuckle out with these clunkers.

One afternoon, a staff member conducting a reading group was on the verge of losing her voice. She passed the dud-filled book to Leonard, one of the residents. Leonard is a retired civil engineer, quietly gregarious by nature and comfortable in group settings. He retains a sharp wit and loves to laugh and to offer pertinent quips. Leonard very helpfully started reading. The group was mesmerized, and convulsed with laughter, for a good half-hour.

I was incredulous, and kept asking if she was sure it had been *that* joke book. She was sure. I tried it the next day and was delighted to observe the same phenomenon. Leonard read the same jokes, quite calmly and simply, and evoked choruses of well-timed, apparently comprehending, laughter. I still don't quite understand it.

One day, after joking and laughing himself into a good mood, Leonard turned toward me, grinning, and said, "You know? If we didn't have a sense of humor, we'd be lost. Of course, sometimes *you're* lost anyway, aren't you? Ha, ha!"

• A Mysterious Story (and Quote) •

Listening to a presentation about some aspect of research on dementia, I was struck by a particular phrase. I wrote it down and approached the speaker afterward to ask if she had been quoting another source or had coined the memorable phrase herself.

With some bewilderment, she shook her head. Not only had she not said what I had written down, but she could not imagine any aspect of her presentation that I could have so misconstrued.

"I'm quite sure. I know I didn't say anything even remotely like that," she assured me, gently shaking her head, probably wondering how many others in her audience had been listening with such imperfect attention.

I kept the quote, though. She liked it, too, whatever its origin:

Laughter unlocks the memories of the heart.

·: 3 :·

Words and Word Games

One of our adult day program clients was enjoying her participation far more than her family had dared hope. "I had a good day," she said one evening, on the ride home. "They talk my language there."

Folks with dementia are a valuable resource for one another. Their efforts to comfort, aid, and reassure one another are legendary. It is thought that less than 10 percent of communication depends on actual words. Still, we use words most of the time, most of our lives. Persons well along their journey with dementia do not necessarily stop using words, but the words change. They often use words, although the words may not be "real."

A great deal has been written about verbal communication with dementia. The following list of dos and don'ts is offered as a distillation of our experience at the A.C.C. in this all-important area.

- Get the individual's attention and keep it; sustain eye contact; use the person's name repeatedly.
- Make sure the individual knows you're there.
  Don't "jump" someone!
- Listen (with all your senses).
  Don't assume you know what an individual has in mind.
- Listen for the real message; match the message (or mood).
  Don't rely on words.

- Give the person time to "get the words out."
  Don't assume that an individual has lost his or her train of thought.
- Supply information in advance.
  Don't ask direct questions.
- Respond to "key" words; "re-feed" partial statements or phrases.
  Don't assume it's all going to be gibberish.
- Use cuing: gestures, facial expressions.
- Use facts; stress the "here and now"; answer the question that is asked.
  Don't reinforce delusions unnecessarily.
- Speak clearly, slowly, and calmly.
- Speak in a low voice, not a loud voice.
- Use simple sentences, one idea at a time.
  Don't use the word *and*.
- Use few words, and words with few syllables.
- Use hackneyed expressions, sayings we've all heard "a million times."
  Don't be afraid to be trite!

• Cognitive Exercise •

Word games, theme-oriented discussions, and reminiscing, provide some of the most useful areas for dementia-appropriate activity. Such activity can be highly effective at home or at a day-care center, in groups or on a one-to-one basis. However, it deals with the two most obvious and challenging areas of dysfunction with dementia: language and memory. There is a fine line between challenge and frustration, between enjoyment and loathing.

The extent to which mental and verbal exercise may serve to slow or ease the progress of dementia is a matter for ongoing research. It appears, though, as with other areas of functioning, that the less we use it, the quicker we lose it. In terms of actual therapeutic progress, the optimistic expectation might be: "Use it, and lose it more slowly, less painfully."

Any cognitive task can seem like a test. Folks will naturally hesitate to participate—to risk failing—unless they are relaxed. In general, a group leader should not call on an individual unless he or she is reasonably sure of receiving a successful reply. Being put on the spot often guarantees a near-panic reflex in any of us, in any group or class situation ("If you hadn't asked me, I could've told you"). Presenting a question or a phrase to the group in general will be less intimidating than calling on an individual directly. The freer folks feel to contribute, the more they will.

One way to get a group to relax is to say, repeatedly, "There is no such thing as a wrong answer" or "Say whatever comes into your head." It is sometimes effective to warn everyone that the next question is very difficult, then ask something quite simple. Above all, the more smiling and good humor in the air, the more relaxed the group will feel.

• Word Games •

Folks with dementia seem to thrive on word games. Any word game should be treated as a separate activity, following the steps outlined in Chapter 1. As always, it is essential that folks be relaxed. A reminder that "any answer is a good answer" or to "say whatever comes to mind" is often helpful. The group leader might ask everyone's help, saying, "I've been getting my mords wixed all morning!"

The group leader might also initiate a discussion of "thing-a-ma-jig-itis": "Do you ever go to say a word, and you can't pull it out? Like, 'Guess who I saw downtown! Good old . . . Oh, you know, good old . . .'" Someone will usually say, "What's-his-name." Another will add, "Who's-it," and so on. Words for things can also be added: "Thing-a-ma-bob," "what-cha-ma-call-it," etc. People with dementia are often in "tip of the tongue" situations. They rise eagerly to this bait, zestfully adding an array of substitute words. The effect appears to be downright cathartic.

The following are examples of specific types of word games, word "warm-ups," or cognitive exercises. None of these lists is exhaustive. Additions to each list are nearly endless, and there are countless additional lists.

The phrases are grouped by word families or grammatical affinities. Using the same type of phrase seems to help folks focus on the task at hand; it helps the activity get rolling (that is, it triggers spontaneous contributions by participants). It is usually best not to mix groups, or families, in any given session. For example, mixing sayings using verbs with sayings using pronouns seems to be jarring to folks. A set of sayings all using, say, the preposition *in* would be somewhat more effective than one using mixed pronouns, and it certainly would be more effective than a hodge-podge list of "hackneyed expressions."

Tongue Twisters

Tongue twisters often work well at the beginning of a cognitive stimulation group. Participants should be encouraged to make mistakes. After all, these are no fun unless we get them mixed up! Copies of the "twister of the day [or week]" may be distributed around the group. Shorter ones might be posted.

1. How much wood would a woodchuck chuck
   If a woodchuck could chuck wood?
   He'd chuck as much wood as a woodchuck could,
   If a woodchuck could chuck wood.

2. Peter Piper picked a peck of pickled peppers.

3. She sells seashells down by the seashore.

4. Big blue rubber baby buggy bumpers.

5. Sister Susie's sewing silken shirts for seven sailors.
   So much skill at sewing shirts our shy young sister shows.
   Still, the sailors send epistles, say they'd sooner sit on thistles
   Than to wear those silken shirts that sister Susie sews!

6. *Pat's Pie.* This developed spontaneously one day, centering on a
   beloved volunteer:
   Pat likes parsnips but not peppers, so she put parsnips, not peppers, in her patented prize potato pie. Pat likes pepper but not paprika, so she sprinkled pepper upon the parsnips but not upon the peppers. Pat put peppered parsnips, not peppers, in her patented prize potato pie!

7. *The Flute Tutor*
   A tutor who tooted the flute
       Tried to tutor two tooters to toot.
           Said the two to the tutor:
           Is it tougher to toot
       Than to tutor two tooters to toot?

8. *Betty Botter's Butter* (Legend has it that this was Sir Lawrence Olivier's vocal warm-up before going on stage.)
Betty Botter bought some butter;
But, she said, "The butter's bitter!
If I put it in my batter,
It will make my batter bitter!"
So she bought some better butter,
Better than the bitter butter,
And she put it in her batter
And her batter was not bitter!
So 'twas better Betty Botter bought some better butter!

9. The Big Blockbuster Blizzard (gleaned from an early-morning weather forecast):
Will we have a big bad blizzard this weekend?

10. This is a zither!

Phrases

There are many uses for the following sets of phrases. The most obvious is simply as a group exercise. Each of the lists can also be made into a worksheet. Worksheets can be valuable as independent activity for those able to do them: some people will actually fill them in, while some may simply read them.

These phrases are among the most automatic, the most used and overlearned, in our language. In fact, many are contained in lists of hackneyed phrases to be avoided! They can ensure success to a wide range of cognitive abilities. The possibilities of role-playing, reminiscing, interpreting, storytelling, and so on, with each phrase are nearly limitless.

The power of automatic sayings and rhymes can last well into the dementia. "These expressions, like music and emotive language, seem to make their way directly into the healthy part of the brain, and are instantly understood . . . probably because of their rhythmic context" (Whitcomb, 1989, p. 28). A common word in each of these sets is the main "trigger"—to speech, what hand-over-hand cuing is to personal care. For example, some folks could complete: "If that's not the pot [calling the kettle black]." Far more automatic, however, would be the same phrase including the main trigger (in this case, the verb): "If that's not the pot calling . . ."

Most phrases offer more than one trigger. "Laughter is the best medicine," for example, is a well-known adage. Some folks could complete "Laughter is . . ." More would be able to complete "Laughter is the . . ." Most would be able to supply the final word: "Laughter is the best . . ."

It is often possible to approach various abilities at nearly the same time. The group leader first gives the most demanding cue, such as, "An apple a day . . ." As some folks more or less successfully complete the saying, the leader can then repeat: "An apple a day keeps the doctor . . ." Merely adding that single, final word often brings a shining smile of achievement.

All such exercises should be introduced by two or three examples. Explanations or rationales need be no more involved than, "I'd appreciate your help to see how familiar these are."

Simple Closure Phrases

The following are basic examples of anomic phrases: they have lost the predicate noun, as so commonly occurs with dementia. Each provides a simple closure exercise. They also illustrate how many of our better-known phrases are song titles.

1. Laughter is the best   [medicine].
2. One bad apple spoils the   [barrel].
3. Another day, another   [dollar].
4. The early bird catches the   [worm].
5. Curiosity killed the   [cat].
6. Keep a civil tongue in your   [head]!
7. As slippery as an   [eel].
8. The cow jumped over the   [moon].
9. A man's home is his   [castle].
10. Don't look a gift horse in the   [mouth].
11. As stubborn as an   [ox].
12. Just as happy as a   [clam].
13. That's the icing on the   [cake].
14. That's water under the   [bridge].
15. "Down by the old mill   [stream]."

16. "I've been working on the   [railroad]."
17. "Let me call you   [sweetheart]!"
18. "Dashing through the   [snow]
    In a one-horse open   [sleigh]."
19. "You are my sunshine, my only   [sunshine]."
20. "Don't sit under the   [apple tree/with anyone else but me]."
21. "Shave and a haircut,   [This common tag, often added to the end of a song, is a very automatic, high-probability cue. Whatever its source, it is old enough to be largely second nature. Individual responses, though, will vary (despite the fact that many individuals without dementia are positive that they know the "right" response). Common variations include "two bits," "bay rum," "shampoo," "close clip," and "pea soup." One musical gentleman with pronounced anomia responds, "Boom, boom!"]."

Fractured Phrases

The previous simple closure phrases and the phrases that follow all lend themselves to "fracturing"; that is, their components can be mixed and matched. Particularly if the phrases are separated by the common word, this can yield surprising results. This provides a fairly active process of straightening out the phrases (and a few laughs). The process also creates frequent repetitions of the phrases. Even the most mentally impaired individuals may become eagerly involved in this, particularly when they feel "in" on the joke.

Sets of cards can be made, small enough for one-to-one use or large enough for use with a group. Naturally, the phrases should be fairly brief for this purpose. ("An apple a day keeps the doctor away" is a bit too long.)

A set of cards might be as follows:

Set A (in black)	*Set B (in red)*
As strong as	an ox
As slippery as	an eel
As wise as	an owl
A memory like	an elephant
As sturdy as	an oak

The black cards would be put up on a board. The red cards might be distributed to the group (with care that they be given to individuals or teams who would not be frustrated by the task and who would not fold, tear, or mutilate them). Or the group leader could simply hold each red card and ask where to put it to make a natural-sounding phrase. The leader might well "mistakenly" place one or more of the red phrases in the wrong place. If placed correctly, the cards might mysteriously become scrambled overnight—or by afternoon.

Verbs

Action phrases are among the most "automatic" of all. If the phrase is presented leaving out only the last word (the terminal noun), then even very cognitively or language-impaired folks can "succeed." The verbs act as triggers. Most of the following sayings become interchangeable if separated between subject and predicate. Examples of "fractured" or non sequitur phrases would be "A new broom . . . keeps the doctor away" or "An apple a day . . . catches the worm."

1. A new broom sweeps   [clean].
2. An apple a day keeps   [the doctor away].
3. A stitch in time saves   [nine].
4. The early bird catches   [the worm].
5. One bad apple spoils   [the barrel].
6. Practice makes   [perfect].
7. Many hands make   [light work].
8. He who laughs last laughs   [best].
9. Bad news travels   [fast].
10. Opportunity knocks   [but once].
11. Absence makes   [the heart grow fonder].
12. One good turn/deed deserves   [another].
13. Time heals   [all wounds].
14. Haste makes   [waste].
15. Slow but sure wins   [the race].
16. Still waters run   [deep].
17. A rolling stone gathers   [no moss].
18. Familiarity breeds   [contempt].

19. Laugh and the world laughs   [with you].
20. He that goes a-borrowing ends up   [a-sorrowing].

Prepositions

Prepositions are among the most frequently used words. They serve to indicate, among other things, position in space: in, out, up, down, under, between, etc. This type of spatial awareness weakens with dementia, especially Alzheimer disease. Regardless of whatever tie-in might be suggested between language and perceptual awareness, the following phrases are very automatic, as well as reaction-provoking. Many lend themselves well to "fractured phrases."

Any prepositions can yield a phrase list. Compiling additional lists is an interesting task that can help give folks good reason to participate.

1. There's nothing new under the   [sun].
2. Water under   [the bridge].
3. A roof over   [our heads].
4. The cow jumped over   [the moon].
5. Plain as the nose on   [his face].
6. The icing on   [the cake].
7. Out of sight, out of   [mind].
8. The handwriting is on   [the wall].
9. Like a fish out of   [water].
10. A needle in   [a haystack].
11. The check is in   [the mail].
12. Don't sit under   [the apple tree].
13. Don't let the cat out of   [the bag].
14. Don't put all your eggs in   [one basket].
15. Don't look a gift horse in   [the mouth].

Similes

Many individuals can work quite independently and enjoyably with fill-in-the-blank tasks such as this. Pencils may be offered.

These phrases were among the first to become "fractured" and remain among the most amusing: "Happy as a cucumber," "Cool as a clam at high tide," etc. There are numerous similes using the word *like*. For whatever reason, these seem a bit more automatic.

1. Happy as a   [clam/clam at high tide/pig in mud/lark].
2. Snug as a   [bug in a rug].
3. Stubborn as a   [an ox/a mule].
4. Nutty as a   [fruitcake].
5. Proud as a   [peacock].
6. Cool as a   [cucumber].
7. Sharp as a   [tack].
8. Flat as a   [pancake/flounder].
9. Busy as a   [bee/beaver].
10. Gentle as a   [lamb].
11. Cute as a   [button/bug's ear].
12. Quiet as a   [mouse].
13. Hard as a   [rock].
14. Smooth as a   [baby's bottom].
15. High as a   [kite].
16. Light as a   [feather].
17. Low as a   [snakes' belly].
18. White as a   [sheet].
19. Pretty as a   [picture].
20. Tall as a   [tree].
21. Clean as a   [whistle].

Triads

There is a special power to the number three. For example, the cue, "One, two, three," is universally helpful in helping folks stand up.

This list of triads is hardly exhaustive; language is full of them. They provide uniquely powerful cuing within themselves. Of all the lists, participants with dementia seem most responsive to these (contributing their own, that is).

The following triads all contain single words. Of course, many familiar triad sayings contain longer phrases, such as "Life, liberty, and the pursuit of happiness," or "The truth, the whole truth, and nothing but the truth," or "Of the people, by the people, and for the people."

Three-word names (Franklin Delano Roosevelt, Martin Luther King, Harriet Beecher Stowe) also fall into this same rhythmic category. With this list, it is especially important to keep age-appropriateness in mind. Many triads that are common today are not automatic for older individuals. Examples of non-age-appropriate triads would be "the good, the bad, and the ugly," "Peter, Paul, and Mary," "Mary Tyler Moore," and "Up, up, and away!"

These also lend themselves especially well to brief anecdotes to set them up. For example: "At a railroad crossing, you might see, stop, look and [listen]." or "Johnny borrowed his dad's car and promised to be home by nine o'clock. When Johnny got home at three a.m., Dad said, 'I want to know where in blue blazes you've been: no ifs, ands, or ____!'"

1. Animal, vegetable, or   [mineral]
2. Every Tom, Dick, and   [Harry]
3. Ready, set,   [Go!]
4. Lock, stock, and   [barrel]
5. Faith, hope, and   [charity]
6. Hook, line, and   [sinker] (not "stinker")
7. Love, honor, and   [obey] (cherish/or trust)
8. Butcher, baker, and   [candlestick-maker]
9. Red, white, and   [blue]
10. Reading, writing, and   [arithmetic]
11. Hip, hip,   [hurray!]
12. Here, there, and   [everywhere]
13. Yesterday, today, and   [tomorrow]
14. Winken, Blinken, and   [Nod]
15. Snap, crackle, and   [pop]
16. Calm, cool, and   [collected]
17. Small, medium, or   [large]
18. Signed, sealed, and   [delivered]
19. Shake, rattle, and   [roll]
20. Ready, willing, and   [able]
21. Morning, noon, and   [night]

Four-Word Phrases

Four-word phrases are noticeably easier for most folks with dementia than three-word phrases. These provide their own special rhythm: one-two, one-two (which may or may not reflect our heart beat).

1. The more,   [the merrier].
2. Easy come,   [easy go].
3. Better late   [than never].
4. Cold hands,   [warm heart].
5. Monkey see,   [monkey do].
6. Like father, [like son].
7. Here today,   [gone tomorrow].
8. Share and   [share alike].
9. Another day, [another dollar].
10. Better safe [than sorry].
11. Live and   [let live].
12. Nothing ventured,   [nothing gained].
13. It's now   [or never].
14. "Swing low, [sweet chariot]."
15. Neither here [nor there].
16. Let bygones [be bygones].
17. Too little, [too late].
18. Easier said [than done].
19. So far,   [so good].
20. It takes   [all kinds].
21. To each   [his own].

Matched Sets

1. Salt and   [pepper].
2. Night and   [day].
3. Bacon and   [eggs].
4. Macaroni and [cheese].
5. Scotch and   [soda].
6. Tea and   [coffee/sympathy/crumpets/cookies/toast].

7. Dogs and   [cats].
8. Back and   [forth].
9. Cake and   [ice cream/pie/coffee/frosting].
10. Needle and   [thread].
11. Sticks and   [stones].
12. Soup and   [sandwich/nuts].
13. Love and   [marriage].
14. Bread and   [butter/water].
15. Soap and   [water].
16. Trick or   [treat].
17. Sink or   [swim].
18. Peace and   [quiet].
19. Shoes and   [socks/stockings].
20. Pins and   [needles].
21. Horse and   [carriage].

Affinities

Many games depend on "trivia" thinking: name such-and-such. This is deductive logic, proceeding from general to specific. Normal trivia-type exercises are poison to people with dementia; this is precisely what they can*not* generally do. An example would be, "Name a brand of cigarettes." Few game-players with dementia would be able to respond to that. Many, though, could answer: "What is a Chesterfield?" Some would quickly say, "cigarette"; some might reply by mimicking the smoking of a cigarette, or by coughing.

1. Fords and Pontiacs are   [cars].
2. Roses and marigolds are   [flowers].
3. Sparrows and robins are   [birds].
4. Boston and Bangor are   [cities].
5. Romeo and Juliet were   [lovers].
6. Maytag and Whirlpool are   [appliances].
7. Harvard and Yale are   [universities].
8. Camels and Winstons are   [cigarettes].
9. T-Bone and porterhouse are   [steaks].

10. Valentino and Gable were   [actors].
11. Sophie Tucker and Kate Smith were   [singers].
12. Squash and cucumbers are   [vegetables].
13. Coke and Pepsi are   [soft drinks].
14. Roosevelt and Eisenhower were   [presidents].
15. Flannel and satin are   [fabrics].
16. Apples and bananas are   [fruits].
17. Trout and bass are   [fish].
18. Pines and maples are   [trees].
19. Vermont and Maine are   [states].
20. Wheaties and Cheerios are   [cereal].
21. Collies and poodles are   [dogs].

There are innumerable other lists of such "things," all of which work well to trigger recall and discussion. The question is, "What is a . . ." or "What does it mean if someone is called a . . ." These may not produce automatic responses, but if participation is voluntary and if the group's atmosphere is good-natured and relaxed, then many folks are likely to offer comments.

Occupations

Occupations can make for good "trivia" questions (What is a . . . ? What does he or she do?).

1. Butcher
2. Carpenter
3. Plumber
4. Pharmacist
5. Astronomer
6. Engineer
7. Secretary
8. Chef
9. Conductor
10. Nurse
11. Chauffeur
12. Valet

13. Lifeguard
14. Meteorologist
15. Ventriloquist
16. Magician
17. Dentist
18. Accountant
19. Milliner
20. Pilot
21. Stenographer

Brand Identification

This exercise is well along the path to "trivia panic." Usually, however, the recognition and reminiscence value of the products named outweighs the difficulty some will have in actually naming the generic item. It is simply fun. It is, nevertheless, one of the most difficult of all the word games sampled here. It points out, like the "affinities" list, the importance of deductive, versus inductive, questions.

While many of these products are still around, they were taken from old magazines (from the 1930s and 1940s) and augmented during group work.

The question is: "What is (or was) . . . ?" An alternative would be, "How do we use . . . ?"

1. Lifebuoy
2. Chase & Sanborn
3. Listerine
4. Maytag
5. Hellman's
6. Ipana
7. Ralston
8. Clorox
9. Aunt Jemima
10. Fletcher's Castoria
11. Pepto-Bismol
12. Fels Naptha

13. Kleenex
14. Odo-ro-no
15. Ovaltine
16. Ken-L-Ration
17. Frigidaire
18. Lydia Pinkham's
19. Texaco
20. Vaseline
21. Gillette

Expletives Deleted

As the story goes, Parson Brown was fixing his fence when he noticed young Johnny, next door, watching his every move with apparent fascination. Finally, the parson said, "Well, Johnny, picking up some pointers on fixing fences?"

"Nope," Johnny replied. "I wanna see what a minister says when he smashes his thumb with a hammer!"

It's amazing how far people will go to "cuss" politely (at least in public). These can be fun and fascinating phrases, but caution is advised! The idea, naturally, is to avoid the swear words.

1. Heavens to   [Betsy/Murgatroyd]!
2. Holy   [Moses/mackerel/Moly/Toledo/Cow/smoke/ Hannah]!
3. Oh, go   [jump in the lake/fly a kite/fry ice/fry an egg/soak your head/take a hike/climb a tree]!
4. Gee,   [(Je)Hoshaphat/whiz/willikers/wizzikers]!
5. As I live and   [breathe/die]!
6. What the   [heck].
7. Oh, for   [heaven's/mercy/goodness/gracious/land's sake]!
8. Oh, my   [Lord/goodness/achin' back/stars and garters]!
9. What in   [Heaven's name/blue blazes/tarnation/the world/ creation]!
10. Son of a   [gun/sea cook/biscuit (limited options but it gets a rise)].
11. Gosh   [darn/Almighty/all fish hooks/all hemlock]!

12. For the love of   [Pete/Mike].
13. Good   [grief/gracious/heavens/Lord/gosh/golly Miss Molly]!
14. Jiminy   [Christmas/Cricket].
15. Jumpin'   [Jerusalem/Jiminy/Jehoshaphat].

Opposites

These can be surprisingly challenging.

1. Up and   [down].
2. In and   [out].
3. Hot and   [cold].
4. Night and   [day].
5. Good and   [bad/evil].
6. Start and   [stop/finish].
7. Beginning and   [ending].
8. Above and   [below].
9. Yes and   [no].
10. Open and   [shut/closed].
11. Long and   [short].
12. Fat and   [slim].
13. Fast and   [slow].
14. Tall and   [short].
15. Smooth and   [rough/scratchy].
16. Rich and   [poor].
17. Bright and   [dark].
18. War and   [peace].
19. High and   [low].
20. Pale and   [ruddy].
21. Generous and   [stingy/miserly/tight/selfish, etc.].

Requests (heard around the house)

1. Turn off the   [lights/heat/TV/stove].
2. Shut the   [door/refrigerator].

3. Use your   [knife and fork/head]!
4. Don't slam that   [door]!
5. Watch your   [step/P's & Q's/mouth]!
6. Do your   [homework/studies/duty]!
7. Wash your   [hands/feet]!
8. Lock the   [door].
9. Please pass the   [salt/sugar/pencil/biscuits/bread and butter].
10. Wash the   [dog/car/dishes].
11. Open a   [window/can of worms].
12. Go take out the   [trash/garbage/rubbish/ashes]!
13. Hang up your   [hat/coat].
14. Go wash behind your   [ears].
15. Go make your   [bed]!
16. Go clean up your   [room]!
17. Go brush your   [teeth/hair]!
18. Put on your   [gloves/mittens/rubbers]!
19. Close the   [door/blinds].
20. Go ask your   [mother/father]!
21. Don't slouch,   [stand up]!

Body Parts

1. You see with your   [eyes].
2. You hear with your   [ears].
3. You kiss with your   [lips].
4. You taste with your   [tongue].
5. You sniff with your   [nose].
6. We have ten   [fingers] and ten   [toes].
7. Comb your   [hair].
8. Go blow your   [nose].
9. Open your   [mouth].
10. Stick out your   [tongue].
11. Brush your   [teeth].
12. Did you wash behind your   [ears]?

13. Raise your   [hand].

14. Clap your   [hands].

15. Wiggle your   [toes].

16. Mittens go on our   [hands].

17. Shoes go on our   [feet].

18. A scarf goes around our   [neck].

19. Ear muffs go on our   [ears].

20. A belt goes around our   [waist].

21. Rings go on our   [fingers].

TV Shows

A very effective phrase-completion exercise with a high probability of success is to use the titles of TV shows. Folks not only are likely to be able to participate, and to enjoy at least passive reminiscing, but also are unusually likely to add names or single-word comments. Our shared TV memory is uniquely well rehearsed.

Folks' recollection of TV shows is far stronger than that of programs from the golden age of radio. Is it because the shows from radio are more distant, and rarely rehearsed, memories? Is it that while radio was in flower for about twenty years, television shows little sign of withering after more than forty years? Is it that television affects (or assaults) two senses to radio's one?

The following list of TV titles is strong in terms of participants' reactions, and they tend to find it very enjoyable. One obstacle is to think of familiar programs with enough words to be self-cuing. Many of the best-recalled shows have single-word titles, (*Gunsmoke, Bonanza*) or feature the stars' names (*The Adventures of Ozzie and Harriet, The Ed Sullivan Show, Alfred Hitchcock Presents*). "Name That Theme Song" games suffer the same failings as *Name That Tune*: some individuals may be able to hum along a bit, but few will do any naming.

Another note: the strongest responses tend to be with the soap operas. Does this reflect increased amounts of time watching daytime television after retirement? Do folks retain some emotional connection to those shows? Is it simply because soaps were/are on the air daily, instead of weekly?

The group leader's additions are limited only by his or her own recollection: Lucy's neighbors' names and some of the foursome's memorable situations, "Come on down" and "It's a new car!" from *The*

Price Is Right, singing *The Ballad of Jed Clampett* (invoking the names of Grannie, Ellie Mae, and Jethro), "The thrill of victory, the agony of defeat" from *Wide World of Sports*, etc., will all be memory joggers.

1. *I Love Lucy*
2. *Days of Our Lives*
3. *The Price Is Right*
4. *The Guiding Light*
5. *The Beverly Hillbillies*
6. *ABC's Wide World of Sports*
7. *The Young and the Restless*
8. *Truth or Consequences*
9. *Father Knows Best*
10. *The Lone Ranger*
11. *Search for Tomorrow*
12. *Have Gun, Will Travel*
13. *Candid Camera*
14. *As the World Turns*
15. *All in the Family*
16. *The Golden Girls*
17. *I've Got a Secret*
18. *The Hallmark Hall of Fame*
19. *Little House on the Prairie*
20. *Leave It to Beaver*
21. *Ted Mack's Original Amateur Hour*

Slogans and Jingles

It's a bit sobering to realize how automatic many advertising slogans have become to us. Many have the extra cuing advantage of being musical (although it's not essential to know the tune).

One of the longest-running advertising slogans—Wisk's "ring around the collar"—should be quite automatic to recall. However, the usual response is *Ring around the Rosie*. Obviously, that saying is even older.

These can often provide moments (or more) of reminiscing as well.

1. I'd walk a mile for a Camel!
2. Maxwell House coffee: Good to the last drop!
3. Wheaties: The breakfast of champions!
4. Winston tastes good, like a cigarette should!
5. That's what Campbell's soups are: Mm, Mm, good!
6. Timex watches: It takes a licking and keeps on ticking!
7. See the U.S.A. in your Chevrolet!
8. Coca-Cola: The pause that refreshes!
9. Clairol: Does she or doesn't she? Only her hairdresser knows for sure!
10. Aren't you glad you use Dial? Don't you wish everybody did?
11. The tiny little tea leaves of Tetley tea!
12. Alka-Seltzer: Ohhh. I can't believe I ate the whole thing!
13. Alka-Seltzer: Plop plop, fizz fizz. Oh, what a relief it is!
14. Let your fingers do the walking (through the Yellow Pages).
15. From the valley of the Jolly (Ho! Ho! Ho!) Green Giant!
16. Ivory Soap: 99 and 44/100% pure—and it floats!
17. Chesterfield cigarettes: Not a cough in a carload!
18. You'll wonder where the yellow went when you brush your teeth with Pepsodent!
19. Morton salt: When it rains, it pours!
20. Bounty paper towels: The quicker picker-upper!
21. Schlitz: The Beer that made Milwaukee famous!

Famous Couples

In the following examples, the individuals with two names tend to be easier: the two names give more clues. For example, "George Burns and Gracie . . ." is easier than "George Burns and . . ."

1. Fred Astaire and Ginger Rogers
2. Nelson Eddy and Jeanette MacDonald
3. Katherine Hepburn and Spencer Tracy
4. Clark Gable and Carole Lombard
5. Mary Pickford and Douglas Fairbanks
6. Lucille Ball and Desi Arnaz

7. Elizabeth Taylor and Richard Burton
8. Roy Rogers and Dale Evans
9. The Lone Ranger and Tonto
10. Fibber McGee and Molly
11. Capt. John Smith and Pocahontas
12. Batman and Robin
13. Tarzan and Jane (Cheetah)
14. Blondie and Dagwood
15. Amos and Andy
16. Adam and Eve
17. Ozzie and Harriet
18. Laurel and Hardy
19. Samson and Delilah
20. David and Jonathan
21. Abbot and Costello

Theme-oriented Exercises

The best discussion topics suggest familiar sayings: proverbs, slogans, jingles, song titles, poems, and so on. Many of these will come spontaneously from participants. A set of ten sayings or songs to start with will often lead to many more.

A few sets of organized closure exercises follow. As with specific topics, these lists can be recycled for many different occasions. In a "theme week," one list could even be used every day and still be challenging, interesting, and fun for most folks. A line from a song may lead to the whole song being sung during the exercise, during a specified sing-along, or both.

"Happy/Grouchy" Stuff

This collection has various applications, such as "smiles," "Cheering up grouches" (as on Monday morning), "rainy days," etc.

1. Laughter is the best   [medicine].
2. Misery loves   [company].
3. Laugh and the world laughs   [with you], weep and you weep   [alone].

4. She is just as happy as a   [clam].

5. He who laughs last, laughs   [best].

6. There's no use crying over spilled   [milk].

7. Always look for the silver   [lining].

8. Laughter does good like a   [medicine].

9. Joy cometh in the   [morning].

10. "Pack up your troubles in your old kit bag and   [smile, smile, smile]."

11. "There'll be bluebirds over the white cliffs of   [Dover]."

12. "When you're smiling, the whole world smiles with   [you]."

13. "Blue skies smilin' at me; nothing but blue skies   [do I see]."

14. "But the smiles that fill my heart with sunshine are the smiles that you give to   [me]."

15. "Every time it rains, it rains pennies from   [heaven]."

16. "Turn your frown upside down, and you will wear a   [smile]."

17. "You'll see the sun come shining through, if you just   [smile]."

18. "Forget your troubles; come on, get   [happy]."

19. "You are my sunshine, my only   [sunshine]."

20. "Gray skies are gonna clear up; put on a happy   [face]."

21. "Smile! You're on   [Candid Camera]!"

Patriotic Stuff

This collection is among the most adaptable, from Veteran's Day to Memorial Day to the 4th of July to V.J. Day to April 18th (Paul Revere's ride). In general, the sayings are (for our purposes) more important than their sources.

1. "Give me liberty, or give me   [death]."

2. "Listen, my children, and you shall hear
    Of the midnight ride of   [Paul Revere]."

3. "One if by land, two if by   [sea].
    And I on the opposite shore will   [be]."

4. "We hold these truths to be self-evident;
    That all men   [are created equal].

That they are endowed by their Creator with certain
Unalienable rights; that among these are
Life, Liberty, and the Pursuit of   [happiness]."

5. Washington: "First in war, first in peace,
    First in the hearts of his   [countrymen]."

6. "'Shoot if you must this old gray head,
    But spare your country's flag!' she   [said]."

7. "From the Halls of Montezuma, to the shores of   [Tripoli]."

8. "Remember the   [Alamo/Maine]."

9. "We'll be over; we're coming over!
    And we won't come back till it's over over   [there]."

10. "Lafayette: We are   [here]."

11. "Uncle Sam wants   [you]."

12. "There'll be bluebirds over the white cliffs of   [Dover]."

13. "Praise the Lord, and pass the   [ammunition]."

14. "December 7th, 1941: A date that will live in   [infamy]."

15. "My Lili of the lamplight; my own Lili   [Marlene]."

16. "Ask not what your country can do for you;
     Ask what you can do for your   [country]."

17. "Oh, beautiful, for spacious skies,
     For amber waves of   [grain]."

18. "God bless America! Land that I   [love]."

19. "Oh, Columbia, the gem of the   [ocean];
     The home of the brave and the   [free]."

Apples

Apples make for a very fertile topic. Here are a few familiar items.

1. Don't upset the apple   [cart].

2. An apple a day keeps the doctor   [away].

3. Her granddaughter is the apple of her   [eye]!

4. New York City is sometimes called   ["The Big Apple]."

5. "Shoo fly pie, and apple   [pandowdy]."

6. One bad apple spoils the   [barrel].

7. That nasty man is rotten to the   [core]!

8. That's like comparing apples and   [oranges].

9. At Halloween, kids bob for   [apples].
10. It's as all-American as Mom and   [apple pie]!
11. A man's voicebox is his Adam's   [apple].
12. They've been riding that old horse; watch your step. The road is full of road   [apples]!
13. "I'll be with you in   [apple blossom time]."
14. "Ida, sweet as apple   [cidah]!"
15. "Don't sit under the   [apple tree]
    With anyone else but   [me],
    Till I come marching   [home]."
16. "With a heart that is true,
    I'll be waiting for you:
    In the shade of the old   [apple tree]."
17. "Ma, I miss your   [apple pie]!
    (And, by the way, I miss   [you, too!])"
18. And never forget: the one thing worse than finding a worm in your apple is finding   [half a worm]!

Chicken and/or Egg

These topics and sayings can be used throughout the year, quite aside from the Easter season.

1. Which came first: the chicken or the   [egg]?
2. Don't put all your eggs in one   [basket].
3. Don't count your chickens before they   [hatch].
4. As scarce as hen's   [teeth].
5. The rooster crows at the break of   [day/dawn].
6. What's good for the goose is good for the   [gander]!
7. Running around like a chicken with its head   [cut off]!
8. "When the (chickens, etc.) come back to   [Capistrano]."
9. Birds of a feather flock   [together].
10. President Hoover promised: "A chicken in every   [pot]!"
11. Why did the chicken cross the   [road]?
12. "Last one in is a rotten   [egg]!"
13. John says his wife nags him; he says he's "hen-   [pecked]."
14. "Oh! The sky is falling in!" said   [Chicken Little].

15. They're on a wild goose   [chase].
16. He's in big trouble; his goose is   [cooked]!
17. One bad egg spoils the   [basket].
18. "A hen is an egg's way of making another   [egg]!"
19. "A chick chick here; a chick chick there;
    Here a chick, there a chick, everywhere a   [chick chick]."

Ben Franklin

Ben Franklin, an amazing character, makes for an interesting group focus. Many sayings (as schoolchildren once knew) are from his *Poor Richard's Almanac*.

1. A bird in the hand is worth two in the   [bush].
2. A penny saved is a penny   [earned].
3. Snug as a bug in a   [rug].
4. Eat to live, not live to   [eat].
5. Little strokes fell great   [oaks].
6. A stitch in time saves   [nine].
7. Where there's marriage without love,
   There will be love without   [marriage].
8. Early to bed and early to rise,
   Makes a man healthy, wealthy, and   [wise].
9. Some are weather wise, some are   [otherwise].
10. Lost time is never found   [again].
11. Remember that time is   [money].
12. Time and tide wait for no   [man].
13. There never was a good war, or a bad   [peace].
14. He that goes a-borrowing, ends up   [a-sorrowing].
15. We never miss the water until the well runs   [dry].
16. Keep your eyes wide open before marriage, half-
    shut   [afterward].
17. Three may keep a secret, if two of them are   [dead].
18. A word to the wise is   [sufficient].
19. God helps those who help   [themselves].
20. Do not squander time, for that's the stuff   [life's made of]!

Cars

Responses to these may vary widely: truly, no answer is a wrong answer.

In a car:

1. You use the windshield wiper to ____.
2. You use the jack to ____.
3. You use the headlights to ____.
4. You use the clutch to ____.
5. You use the gas pedal to ____.
6. You use the brake to ____.
7. You use the horn to ____.
8. You use the seatbelt to ____.
9. You use the map to ____.
10. You use the mirrors to ____.
11. If you see a red light, you ____.
12. If you see a green light, you ____.
13. If you see a school, you ____.
14. If you see a stop sign, you ____.
15. If you see an ambulance, you ____.
16. If you need gas, you ____.
17. If you come to a toll booth, you ____.
18. If you see a moose in the road, you ____.
19. If your car breaks down, you ____.
20. If you see a hitch-hiker, you ____.
21. If you come to a railroad crossing, you ____.

• Discussions •

A directed discussion of a specific topic may be the heart of a cognitive stimulation group. The idea is to stimulate and gather ideas, impressions, words, and memories from the group and to blend them into a shared experience.

It is important to recall the limitations of mere words. We gather memories through all our senses. Recall is triggered by all the senses, often in combination. Therefore, the multisensory approach is always helpful. Talking and singing about apples is fine; holding, feeling, and eating an apple is likely to be more effective.

Many individuals have a dominant sense: one that they pay the most attention to, one through which they filter the bulk of their experience. If my dominant sense is smell, then odors will tend to trigger more sensation, more memory for me, than sounds.

More important for present purposes, though, may be the sensory losses common in dementia, especially decreased acuity in smell and taste. Sensory losses secondary to normal aging are also significant: losses in hearing, visual acuity, and touch sensitivity, as well as smell and taste.

A group discussion does not need to be a long, complex affair: a good fifteen-minute session is great. Forty-five minutes may be too long, if only because the less verbal participants may have wandered away. Too, by then everyone will welcome a respite from the group leader's voice.

The most important thing for the group leader is to have a good topic and questions about it. To have questions, the leader needs only to think of the five W's of journalism: who, what, why, when, where (and sometimes how). Using these simple triggers, he or she can create a discussion around almost any object or topic, anytime and anywhere. In a way, this is fundamental social or "cocktail party" thinking. Enough questions can be easily generated, whether the topic is dogs, George Washington, or a pencil. The goal is to unlock knowledge or comments by the participants, not the leader. Anyone with an imperfect memory would do better to write down the questions in advance. A "baker's dozen" of questions is usually plenty.

The ploy of playing dumb is often helpful: "Gee, does anyone know what this is?" Being "much too young [or old]" can also lend an ironic note of help for a group leader.

Another useful stimulus is the key-word approach: "What words come to mind when you hear this?" or "What do you think of when you hear . . . ?" Although this is an open-ended approach, it need not create undue stress unless an individual participant is singled out (called on) to respond. Individuals' word associations are fascinating. Each word can be added to a list, and provide an additional key word trigger.

Nothing can be more valuable to a group leader than training in the traditional basic remotivation technique (see Appendix D). Much of what follows contains echoes of this tried, true, and effective method of planning and conducting group work. As with all aspects of dementia work, new and adaptive wrinkles are required.

Discussion topics should be:

- Objective and concrete (as with remotivation guidelines). Discussions should center around people, not feelings; objects, not concepts. "Women" might be appropriate; "Mother" might not. The American flag might be fine; "patriotism" could be slippery.
- Specific. "Women" might be effective; "nurses" might be better. The director of nursing, now making her entrance in whites, with cape and cap, hot water bottle and mustard plaster in hand, might be that much better. "Fruit" might get some mileage, but "apples" would get more; talking about apples and then making a pie together would be better yet, and would mirror one of the most common of all remotivation groups.
- Familiar (age-appropriate). The topic should be generally familiar to the group: something that "most of us" have known about at some point and are interested in. If the topic is of general knowledge, then it will almost automatically be of interest.
- Available. Materials relating to the topic should be readily available: the more, and the more varied, the better.

The most effective topics tend to involve icons: that is, pictures or visual images that people generally recognize, that have an almost magical cultural significance. These include people, events, music, technological developments, foods, fads, and social and religious customs. Special icons for folks now elderly include pictures of George Washington, Abraham Lincoln, F. D. and Eleanor Roosevelt, Amelia Earhart, Uncle Sam, Shirley Temple, Laurel and Hardy, Bing Crosby, and Kate Smith. "Nonpeople" icons include the American flag, Coca-Cola (bottles and logos), the Model T, the RCA dog, and so on. It is important for all caregivers to familiarize themselves with these generational icons.

The best topics include connections with familiar sayings or songs. They also lend themselves to humor; reminiscing; slogans; demonstrations or hands-on manipulation; food or beverage tie-ins; related videos, pictures, posters, or other audiovisuals. (As I write this, a candle, a light bulb, and an old Victrola are being used in a birth-date discussion of Thomas Edison—a "grade B" topic at best. Pictures include Edison himself, light bulb advertisements, the G.E. logo, movie posters, and old RCA Victor ad featuring the dog listening to "his master's voice.")

Mention of upcoming holidays is also traditional discussion fare. Historical events or birth dates of famous people and residents can provide discussion material and reinforcement of time orientation. These can be brief or can take an hour. Many almanacs and calendars contain such "day-to-day" information and can be invaluable in suggesting topics. Some helpful almanacs:

Brennan, Jim. *Jim's Special Events Calendar and Planning Guide (1994)*. Brennan Associates, 237 Springfield St., Wilbraham, MA 01095–2226, (413) 596–2525

Chase's Annual Events: The Day by Day Directory (published yearly). Chicago: Contemporary Books, Inc. Available in reference sections of most libraries.

Daily Planet Almanac (1985). New York: Avon Books/Daily Planet, Inc.

On This Day: A collection of over 8,000 events for every day of the year (1992). Avenel, N.J.: Crescent Books/Reed International Books, Ltd.

Certain very familiar topics may trigger powerful thoughts and memories of a negative, disturbing nature. Examples would be the *Titanic*, the *Hindenburg*, the Depression, Pearl Harbor, John F. Kennedy's assassination, and the Vietnam conflict. While such topics need not be avoided altogether, they should certainly be handled with care.

Some sure-fire discussion topics—concrete, specific, familiar, and available—have been:

1. George Washington
2. Abraham Lincoln
3. Franklin D. Roosevelt
4. Bing Crosby
5. Tea and/or coffee
6. Apples

7. Tomatoes
8. Bread
9. Strawberries
10. Chocolate
11. School days (especially in September and June)
12. Moose (the existence of which proves that the Creator has a sense of humor)
13. Chickens (and/or eggs)
14. Colds and flu (especially in season)
15. Soup
16. Patent/herbal medicines
17. Ice/ice cream (especially therapeutic during heat waves)
18. Bears (including Teddies)
19. "Our" state
20. Automobiles (old cars/Model T)
21. Smiles (grouches and how to cheer them up!)

Elements for a sample discussion follow. The topic is molasses, a good-but-not-great topic. It is familiar to older folks, and it lends itself to some nostalgia and reminiscing. There are some obvious tie-ins with food, language, and music, and some props are easy to come by. There just isn't a lot of anything: it's a relatively limited subject. It might not be suitable as a "theme of the week," but can make for a good fifteen-minute session.

I like to haul this out in January, to commemorate the Great Boston Molasses Flood of 1919. The event itself is not necessarily cheerful; there were twenty-one casualties and several horses perished. It requires handling with kid gloves and it certainly is not an event to be dwelt on in detail. The following suggestions, while not exhaustive, have developed from a number of groups over several years.

Molasses

Materials to have on hand:

- Brief encyclopedia entries about molasses.
- Recipes from the old "Fannie Farmer" cookbook.
- Props such as:

—A bottle of rum

—An old jug, such as would have been used to store molasses.

—Current containers of molasses

—A can of sugar cane

—A package of store-bought molasses cookies

- Questions, such as:

    —What is (What do you think when you hear) molasses?

    —Please help me spell molasses (as a display/poster).

    —What does molasses look like (color, consistency, etc.)? Demonstrate pouring it.

    —Where does molasses come from? Briefly use the researched information.

    —Are there different types of molasses? (Folks may recall black strap, etc.)

    —What does molasses taste like? (Offer samples in small medicine cups.)

    —How do we use molasses? (On foods, e.g., pancakes, pudding; in ginger snaps; in taffy and taffy "pulls.")

- Traditional, more or less automatic sayings:

    —Slow as cold molasses (in January)

    —A traditional spring tonic was sulphur and molasses (or molasses and onions).

- Offer samples of the store-bought molasses cookies. Most tasters will decide that these are definitely inferior to what Grandma used to make. It will probably be necessary to bake a batch of "real" molasses cookies (for which the kitchen might plan to supply the basic dough). These could then be served as a snack, for tea, or for a dessert. A daiquiri party would be another option.

- Traditional molasses songs:

    I don't know any either, aside from *Rum and Coca-Cola*, although Spike Jones did have a popular recording called, *Molasses*, which is still amusing. Molasses is, however, sweet; if the field is enlarged to include "sweet" songs, then the variety is nearly unlimited. A few examples include: *Let Me Call You Sweetheart, Love's Old Sweet Song, When You Were Sweet Sixteen, Ida, Sweet as Apple Cidah, Sweet Georgia Brown, Goodnight,*

*Sweetheart, Ain't She Sweet, The Sweetheart of Sigma Chi, Sugar
Time, In the Sweet By and By,* and so on.

Finding materials for a discussion is often a process of ingenuity. Many
specific objects create their own discussions: a dog, a baby, a horse, a
running antique car, or a working, science-project volcano. Other
sources can include:

- New and old magazines. Older magazines tend to be much
  larger in size than new ones, and to make a better display.
  Older advertising, besides being "old fashioned," tends to
  use simpler art than is common today. Some items, then and
  now, tend to be heavily promoted in advertising: pineapple
  used to be, for example. In modern magazines, it is amazing
  how many ads feature strawberries.
- The nearest supermarket. Shopping can yield a surprising
  wealth of items related to a theme: strawberries, blueberries,
  chocolate, eggs.
- Supermarket suppliers. The companies who supply the produce, for example, also supply advertising materials: posters,
  brochures, pictures.
- Yard sales and flea markets
- The Yellow Pages
- "Learning" stores. (The toy stores with the pricey German toys.)
  Many such stores feature "teacher's rooms" that have a great
  array of educational materials, many highly appropriate in
  terms of both specific topics and cognitive ability.
- Remnant/liquidation stores
- Salvation Army and other thrift stores. (Browsing will some-
  times yield unsuspected topics, such as ugly ties.)
- State agencies. Potentially valuable materials can be obtained
  from such state agencies as (in Maine) the Sardine Council,
  the Milk Commission, the Agriculture Promotion Office, the
  Publicity Bureau, etc.
- "Party goods" stores (especially for paper products)
- Local social studies and science teachers

"Name That Thing"

When we first opened, I had high hopes for using "busy boxes." They seemed like an ideal solution for a number of difficult situations. If an individual was anxious, then we could pass him or her a box full of individually chosen items. These might be specially selected and kept on hand for the specific individual, or they could be objects chosen for "sure-fire" fascination for anyone. The presumption was that the person would rummage through the contents of the box, thereby decreasing his or her anxiety and diverting the focus from a problem behavior (such as pillaging another resident's room or trying to tear apart a window at 3:00 A.M.).

This approach rapidly proved to be less than practical. A "busy box," in itself, usually required one-to-one help to connect the individual's attention to one or more objects within. It was no more effective (and often less so) than any other appropriate individual or busy work type of activity, presented on a one-to-one basis. A "busy" drawer, presented to a woman bent on pillaging dresser drawers, simply became one more drawer. A substitute dresser (in a quiet place, away from the bedrooms) rarely proved diverting for long. Moreover, busy boxes proved to be a housekeeping nightmare. The benefit to individuals rarely outweighed the mess and clutter, not to mention the staff time needed to clean up and rearrange each box.

Despite this disappointment, though, several beneficial developments came from the busy-box experiments. Our activity closet (which is located in our living room area and is generally kept locked) serves as a giant busy box. When an individual needs diversion, an array of possibilities can be found in there; one will usually work. (See Table and Social Activities, Chapter 4.)

Individuals' reactions to such boxes suggested a group box type of format.

The box itself is a cube-shaped ($2' \times 2' \times 2'$) plastic storage container with a lid. It's red, simply to attract attention. One or more objects—generally simple, familiar items—are placed in the box. It is used much like the traditional "What's in the bag?" type of activity, often in one-to-one or in-room work. It can be effective with small groups and even with circle groups of twenty-odd people.

The items in the box are revealed one at a time, either by the group leader or by "daring" members of the group. The first step is to name the thing. The "no answer is wrong" rule is always important. Participants may well offer descriptive words rather than actual labels (for example, imitation crowing rather than "rooster").

Each item may trigger some discussion: What does this put you in mind of? Is this real? What color would you call this? What shape is it? Would you have this in your house? What do you think of when you see one of these? Where would you find one of these? What's the French word for this?

Items may be passed around the group. (Usually, though, no item will ever make it all the way around a group; someone will fancy it and keep it. The larger the group, the more likely this is.) Common items in our box include: a plastic (lawn ornament) chicken; a rubber chicken ("lunch"); a washboard; a flatiron; bars of soap; a football; a baseball mitt (antique or modern); plastic fruit; plastic flowers; hand puppets; funny hats; a plastic flamingo (which very few participants with dementia have ever been able to name, instead calling it a swan, pelican, duck, or even "that damned thing with the crooked neck"). The possibilities are endless.

If a limited number of items are presented, they could then be used for various short-term memory games. The simplest of these is to wait a few minutes, then ask for guesses as to what had been in the box. It may be a good idea to announce this in advance: "In a few minutes, we'll see if anyone recalls any of the things." If short, descriptive words are attached to each item—such as "the plastic (rooster)," "the beautiful new (floppy felt hat)"—it will aid some individuals to recall the item or to be secure enough with their recollection to take a guess. It may aid recollection to return the items to the box in the same order in which they came out.

If the box is used daily, then items may be added each day: say, two or three on Monday, the same items plus one more on Tuesday, and so on. A total of five items to show, discuss, and fondle is usually sufficient in any case. The items may reflect traditional aspects of each day: washboard on Monday, flatiron on Tuesday, rubber fish on Friday.

Asking the group to guess what items might be in the box creates a relatively high-pressure situation, and many individuals may hesitate to do so. Others, though, will leap at the chance to show off. The usual aids to relaxation will help maintain a feeling of comfort: not asking individuals directly, praising any statements, making all answers "right," and, above all, keeping the whole thing in good humor, as more or less a joke. For individuals who participate verbally, this exercise can provide a very informal gauge of short-term recall and learning ability.

Not surprisingly, some folks do learn a given item through a week's presentation from the box. Their recall, however, is often better after a weekend: they may recall more on Monday than they had the previous Friday. It's helpful to have a box full of items in case someone randomly recalls one from last Tuesday or from a month ago.

One lady was intrigued by a shapeless, black, felt "character" hat. She would usually "model" it with the same mugging. However, she never actually anticipated it. Eventually, the hat vanished. Months later, one morning, as the box was being explored, she said, "There might be a hat." I explained where the hat had gone, but she rarely failed to predict that the hat was in the box. Then the hat reappeared (I rarely know where things reappear from). She regularly predicted the hat for years afterward.

• Readings •

A reading is a special type of discussion group. It is similar to what the word implies, whether a Saturday morning kiddies' story hour at the library or radio story program, but adapted for dementia. Mainly, the readings consist of various short segments: a melange, a patchwork quilt of short, sweet bits.

A daily reading group has been a staple since our opening day, when a well-meaning staff member discovered that folks were not enthralled by A. A. Milne's poetry. (Most Maine parents of several generations ago did not read *When We Were Six* to their kids, and by and large could not have heard it in their own childhoods, as Mr. Milne had not yet begun producing his famed works.) Originally, I used the term "reading" simply for want of a better label. It's really a bit of a misnomer: there's usually a lot more storytelling than actual reading, and often a lot more singing than anything else.

The group is held in a quiet, intimate, and relatively secluded room. Many of our staff members and volunteers much prefer this setting to the morning, dining-room/living-room setting. Above all, there is less distraction or background noise than in the wide-open space of the main room. There are also fewer human distractions (staff, nonparticipating residents, visitors, etc.). The room itself (by design) has a relaxed, tranquil feel to it. One's voice is an easier instrument to play in this setting.

Just as the higher-energy programs lend themselves to the morning hours, this lower-key session lends itself to afternoon or evening. Its usual position in our daily routine serves many functions, not the least of which is to mask the inevitable coming-and-going of shift change. (Although our staffing schedule does include some staggered shift assignments, there is still a significant—and potentially catastrophic— change at three o'clock: "My God, everybody's going-going-gone home. I'd better go too!"

The so-called reading group usually runs from (more or less) 2:30 P.M. to (more or less) 3:30 P.M. When folks emerge from the group, they basically see familiar staff faces. They tend not to realize that the familiar faces are different.

In terms of numbers, this is sometimes the largest group activity of the day, excepting meals. Similar groups are frequently conducted, although with fewer participants, and for shorter periods, as needed. A group is generally held in the evening, at roughly 6:30.

Along with a wide range of mental and social stimulation, readings provide a component of relaxation. Reading and listening are in themselves relaxing, or at least can be. Many of us retain early-learned patterns of reading before falling asleep. (One resident still had to fall asleep with a book in her hand: reading, even though the book was upside down). Many folks (whether going to bed at night, going *back* to bed at night, or lying down for a nap after lunch) still benefit from a little quiet chat once they're tucked in; others benefit from soft songs, even lullabies, before they drift away.

It is rare that at least one person doesn't sleep during a reading. The only problem, assuming that day-napping is not contraindicated for the individual, is if the snoring becomes deafening. We often count it a success when a given individual actually catches a catnap. He or she is usually not one of those who will lie down and take a much-needed siesta.

I occasionally conduct readings with the intent of inducing rest, if not actual mass somnolence. An example of this would be after returning from an outing. It may look a bit odd, but it is very helpful for those verging on "rest deprivation." (Longfellow's *Song of Hiawatha*, read unedited and stressing the singsong rhythm, is especially useful for this. Songs such as *Sweet and Low* or *Love's Old Sweet Song* can also be helpful.)

Sleep is not, however, the overall goal of most readings. I have seen more miracles in the reading setting than in any other, including one-to-one sessions: moments of real reminiscing by normally nonverbal folks; flashes of shocking short-term recall; witty wisecracks; wonderfully awful puns; pearls of knowledge and wisdom from individuals usually unable, or hesitant, to contribute in a group or "public" setting.

A reading is quite easy to do effectively. It is also quite easy to do unsuccessfully. The basics are similar to those for any other activity (see the steps in a structured activity described in Chapter 1). The physical setup of the room is crucial. The shape of our room dictates an oval, which is basically very good. However, anyone who cannot see the reader(s) or group leader(s) is likely to be uninvolved. Some whose ability to participate in morning discussion or sing-alongs is limited by impaired hearing or sight may be able to join the reading with great success if they sit close to the reader(s).

The position of the group leader can be especially important; the leader will generally work the crowd with voice and eye contact only. In our situation, the group leader does best to sit in the back of the room, away from the doors that lead to and from the main hallway. This tends to attract the group's attention away from goings-on in the corridor. The back of the room is also the turnaround point for wanderers; the group leader is then ideally placed to assist those who wander in to either join the group or wander back out again. Other individuals do better sitting with their backs to the windows along one wall. Then they do not offer a running commentary on the various trucks and cars coming and going, the movement of tree branches in the wind, various cats peering in the window, and so on.

As always, preparation is essential. It is not advisable to "wing" a reading. I try to at least skim-read anything I plan to use. Ad-libbing with a few folks for a few minutes is one thing; ad-libbing with twenty-five people for an hour is another. Some basic breathing or relaxation exercises can be very useful in setting a restful, attentive, mood.

We start with a song. This can be at random or by choice. I like to present an individual with several bunched-together songbooks, or a sheaf of music, or one book, and ask him or her to open it up, anywhere at all. We then sing the song, and all its verses, if we know it. If we don't know the piece, then it often makes an intriguing poem, possibly quite comical. Some selectivity is in order. For example, the pages containing *Home Sweet Home* and *M.O.T.H.E.R.* have long been "edited out."

We usually sing at least one song that everybody knows. This sometimes takes a few minutes and sometimes lasts for the entire session. Some folks depart after this musical phase. Some, naturally, depart after fifteen minutes, whether or not the singing has concluded.

The most vital dynamic of this group is the frequency of breaks in whatever is being read. These breaks refocus attention that may have wandered. Questions or comments about the material, often from a participant, will provide an appropriate break.

While it would seem that the incremental repetition inherent in a novel, or even a short story or article, read day to day, would be effective, it just doesn't tend to work that way. For people with dementia, the memory loss is generally too profound.

Options for a short reading include:

- Familiar (short) poems
- Nonthreatening trivia quizzes
- Brief items of interest. The *National Enquirer* is an especially good source. Weekly items such as *Why I Love My Pet, Happy Thoughts,* and *What Happened Last Week* are ideal, as are numerous brief, positive, heart-warming, amusing, or intriguing bits.

  It is important to distinguish between the *National Enquirer* and most other tabloids. Nowadays the *National Enquirer* contains mostly news and celebrity gossip; it does not usually carry such lurid features as *Bigfoot Ate My Children,* or *My Children Ate Bigfoot,* or worse. Of course, most current celebrities are about as interesting to folks with dementia as silent film stars would be to teenagers.

- Songs or tidbits played on a cassette player, for singing along or brief listening. Old radio shows (comedy routines, program introductions, or advertisements) can be effective—usually in short segments.

Options for a longer reading include:

- A *very* short story
- A short chapter from a novel or other book (especially if related to a special theme)

- An article or other piece from a periodical. Many of our most successful pieces have come from *Good Old Days, Reminisce,* and *Reader's Digest.*
- A story told (recalled, made up, etc.). These can be real anecdotes or obviously tall tales. Storytelling can have a place of great value here, as elsewhere. Some very good stories are all the better for being paraphrased and read or told in the first person, as if they actually happened to the reader.
- The *Soap Opera News* (plot synopses) from the *National Enquirer.* These make great dramatic reading—the more mock serious, the better.
- Certain discussion topics seem especially suited to this format. Examples include participants' nicknames and middle names.

A special value of familiar poetry is that folks will tend to recite together. There was a time in American education when children memorized poems by rote. Our folks remember a surprising amount of snippets.

It's largely the same dynamic as singing *Let Me Call You Sweetheart:* familiarity breeds comfort. The sort of poem learned in childhood has reminiscent value as well, on a far more nonverbal level.

Many, if not most, children's poems are well recalled, though potentially tricky to introduce. Good examples include *Winken, Blinken, and Nod, The Duel, The Owl and the Pussycat,* and many Mother Goose rhymes.

Especially good poems (in the sense of being effective) are:

1. *Trees,* by Joyce Kilmer (universally known if not admired)
2. *Stopping by Woods on a Snowy Evening,* by Robert Frost
3. *Home,* by Edgar Guest
4. *Little Things,* by Julia Fletcher
5. *Do It Now,* Author unknown
6. *A Visit from St. Nicholas,* by Clement Moore (year round; refreshing in a July heat wave)
7. *The Modern Hiawatha,* by George A. Strong
8. *The Arrow and the Song,* by Henry Wadsworth Longfellow
9. *The Village Blacksmith,* by Henry Wadsworth Longfellow

10. *Paul Revere's Ride,* by Henry Wadsworth Longfellow (Selected portions; apparently no one has ever learned the whole thing and it gets tedious in the middle. But everyone knows the beginning and the end!)
11. *The Town of Don't-You-Worry,* by I. J. Bartlett
12. *There Was a Little Girl,* sometimes attributed to Longfellow
13. *Casey at the Bat,* by Ernest Lawrence Theyer

Most verses to songs can serve as poems, with the well-known chorus sung or recited by all. Examples include: *After the Ball, The Man on the Flying Trapeze, Daisy, Daisy (Daisy Bell),* and *Yes! We Have No Bananas!*

Many psalms are familiar and overlearned; all are beautiful.

Spelling can be part of any discussion group. Some individuals love to spell; often, these folks are very good spellers. Others may be seen mouthing letters silently. I like to make signs or posters with a group—partly to save time but also to encourage group spelling. (It's especially believable to "play dumb" when spelling.) Spelling bees, however, provide a good example of what not to do in a dementia setting. Group spelling can be effective—and invites participation—when it is relaxed, which is to say voluntary. Even if individuals are not called on during a spelling bee, they may very well spell a word incorrectly, and others are likely to notice. In an informal setting, such as making a sign, that could be de-emphasized; in a formal, "bee" setting, a mistake is out there for all to hear.

Several precautions pertain to the conclusion of these groups. First, some folks will be a bit unsteady after sitting for so long. Singing a "walking" song, or just stamping feet for a few moments, may help.

We sometimes depart singing a song, alerting the staff that we're "on our way." Twenty-odd people suddenly surging out into the hall can create chaos. Given the time of day and the possible fatigue of certain individuals, special vigilance is necessary to ensure a safe and smooth transition to the next activity (as, in the late afternoon, to a social, food-oriented activity). One resident, if left on her own during this transition, would invariably confront some individual and rapidly fly into a catastrophic rage. If escorted, however, she would with equal reliability make the transition with her cheerful and secure mood intact.

• A Good Idea with Mixed Results •

A student volunteer once offered to conduct a relaxation/visualization therapy session. This volunteer was enrolled in a professional undergraduate program and had excellent credentials. It certainly sounded like a worthwhile idea. It seemed especially promising for two residents, Aggie and Bonnie, who typically became overly tired during the afternoon and resisted encouragement to rest in any formal way.

The group was conducted during our after-lunch Quiet Hour. A group of about eight was assembled. I checked on proceedings after about five minutes. Two participants had departed, but things seemed to be going well. When I checked in again, about fifteen minutes later, several individuals were, in fact, sound asleep, and Aggie was among them.

Bonnie, however, seated within eye-shot of the door, put a finger to her lips, signaling me to be silent, and nodded toward the group leader. The leader was the most relaxed slumberer of all.

• An Innovative Program Concept •

A problem was developing. As fall progressed and our program shifted from summer to autumn, it became clear that a high anxiety/agitation level was developing between the end of breakfast and the beginning of the exercise group. This period, more or less a half an hour, had been a fairly tranquil, social period through summer. It was far too long a lull, now.

I began to search my memory for a solution that was not a reading, was not musical, was not exercise, was not task oriented: that is, something different. The modality would have to be a core group program; one that required minimal development and preparation; one that could be conducted, with minimal training, by a variety of caregivers, during the week and on weekends (no one on staff cared to commit to an additional group activity, daily, at 9:30 A.M.); and one that, given the hour, was fairly low-key. I wanted something unique, to boot.

A few mornings later, the head nurse patiently asked if I had come up with such an idea. I had to admit that I had not. In fact, the more I'd cogitated, read, and talked with staff members, the more questions I had identified.

"Well, they need something," the head nurse said. "How soon were you going to start the exercise group?"

"In about fifteen minutes," I replied. "I could start now, I guess."

"No, no," she said. "Finish what you were doing. I'll just sit down with the newspaper. I was going to take a break and read the paper anyway."

So she did. And she just happened to start reading the personal ads in the classified section: *Talking Personal: Meet a New Friend — or a New Love!* I went to find out what was triggering such gales of laughter, such lucid and spontaneous participation by so many individuals.

Truly, there is little new under the sun. So often, the best solutions are the most simple, the most obvious: how many of us depend on a good dose of the morning newspaper? And how few folks with dementia can really enjoy it independently anymore?

The morning paper has been a daily staple since then. We do shy away from "hard" news and most actual "current events," which tend to be bewildering, if not frightening, to folks with dementia.

Enjoyable group subjects tend to be such features as, first and foremost, the weather (including the previous day's high and low temperatures nationally); *Today's Chuckle* (which can continue to gather chuckles, repeatedly, all day); community events, meetings, and programs (school lunch menus and public suppers make for great reading); Ann Landers and Dear Abby (with discretion); and horoscopes. Human-interest stories are often winners, although, as with the *National Enquirer,* most featured celebrities are largely unknown to folks with dementia. Advertising fliers are often intriguing. Any supermarket flier can create an instant *The Price Is Right* session; seasonal fliers can provide convenient decorations.

Comics can often be put to good use. Some comic strips often feature old jokes (especially *B.C., Frank and Ernest,* and *Shoe,* among others). *Blondie* not only has punchlines that are frequently funny but also has the added benefit of familiarity, having been around since the 1920s. *The Family Circus* is often good for cuteness. *The Far Side* is usually beyond the ken of a person with dementia, to say the least. "Serious" strips, such as *Mark Trail,* can make for extremely dramatic (if slow-moving) reading day-to-day.

The newspaper is used for folks to peruse individually or on a one-to-one basis. Either way, the plain old daily newspaper is good stuff.

·: 4 :·

Table and Social Activities

As in many "real" homes, the A.C.C.'s structured activities most often occur at the dining-room tables. Especially in the early afternoon, the dining room tends to be a quietly busy workroom.

• Table Activities •

It would be quite feasible to organize the bulk of the programing around table activities, as some adult day centers do. The main deterrent is that such an approach tends to be labor-intensive. Where a team of two could well conduct an hour's large-group programing, six "busy" tables might require a team of four or five, if not one helper per table.

The following activities are also useful in other areas (office, kitchen) and for individuals not involved in group programs. Work-oriented and diversionary, they range from one-to-one (though rarely independent as such) to small-group activities, depending on the task and how many chairs can fit around the table.

Separate tables will almost automatically be graded by skill level. If a task arrayed on a table is attractive—that is, if it looks "doable"— then folks will tend to be engaged by it. Individuals will tend not to stay with a task that is overwhelming.

If puzzles of varying levels of mental skill are arrayed on the tables, individuals will tend to gravitate toward the puzzle that is most cognitively appropriate for them. This type of activity can often be self-motivating or self-involving. Items left for individuals to discover at 2:00 A.M. or in a "busy" area are examples of this. Of course, the items should never be dangerous or valuable, or likely to be eaten or thrown.

Extending a specific task can often be easily accomplished by sleight-of-hand. For example, to extend the task of folding laundry, the staff helpers will reach into the laundry cart and undo what was just done, producing yet more items to fold. Items that have been sorted can also be "unsorted" and presented anew.

The following activities usually require minimal preparation and setup time. Individuals may need a bit of assistance to get involved or to remain so. A given task might not be inviting in and of itself, but the request to "help"—for example, to "see if all the pieces are there"—might well be.

We keep most "busy" materials in a centrally located closet. They are loosely organized by the nature of the individual tasks: winding, sorting, puzzles, manipulative, and so on. The knowledge of an individual's abilities, history, likes and dislikes, and present mood dictates what specific items might be selected. As a rule, one of three appropriate tasks will work with a given individual at a given moment on a given day. In other words, take out three, and the odds are that one will be effective.

Complaints such as "I just folded that basket of things!" are rare. But the same task cannot always be repeatedly presented within the same day or hour. With more lucid individuals, a given task should not be offered more than every other day; with some, once a week.

One hallmark of success with "busy" activity materials is their disappearance. The more engaging a task, the more likely the items are to be hoarded, to emerge eventually from someone's drawer, purse, or closet.

A Baker's Dozen of Table Activities

Many of the following items are commercially available. The number after some items corresponds to the number in the list of catalogs provided as Appendix D. Some items may be carried by more than one catalog; the number merely indicates the one from which we happened to order.

1. Simple Magazine Browsing
   Newer issues are preferable to older ones for browsing. (Aside
      from the possible disorienting impact of out-of-date publica-
      tions on the residents, it is disconcerting, at the least, for visi-
      tors to find residential facilities littered with years-old maga-
      zines.)

2. Magazine Scavenger Hunt
   The aim here is for people to find a picture in a magazine of the
      item or subject that has just been named. The item being
      searched for should be specific and objective, following the
      guidelines for discussion topics. It is sometimes helpful to
      place a card with the subject written on it (e.g., "dogs" or
      "apples") on display in the middle of the table.
         Pictures found can be saved for group discussions, glued
      onto separate sheets of paper or cardboard, onto "cheer up"
      or birthday cards, or into a collage.
         In such a directed activity, old magazines—especially very
      old or reminiscent issues—can be particularly useful.

3. The Round Wooden Puzzle (catalogs 12 and 14)
   Actually assembling our round wooden puzzle—it lacks a pic-
      ture and is not color coded—is a rather complex enterprise
      (for any of us!). Working at it, however, is often quite engag-
      ing. As with any puzzle, the "purpose" (not wholly fictitious)
      may be to "see if all the pieces are here." It fits neatly onto,
      and is nearly the size of, our dining room tables. The pieces
      of this puzzle are among the most independently manipu-
      lated—and hoarded—of all our "busy" objects.

4. The Giant Animal Puzzle (catalog 2)
   The giant animal puzzle is exactly that: measuring three feet
      square, it covers an entire table and has pictures of common
      farm animals and their young. The pieces are large, simple,
      and not especially infantile.

5. Almost any puzzle of the United States

6. Towels
   In addition to the facility linen, which folks work on at least ev-
      ery other day, we often keep one or more baskets of used
      "household" towels. We periodically solicit donations, how-
      ever old or tattered. These can be brought out for endless
      folding (and unfolding and refolding). One drawback to this

task is that it sometimes becomes very territorial: "Touch my towels and I'll deck you!"

7. Spools/Ropes/Knots

One of the most routine motions is winding. It can provide many engaging types of tasks. The most traditional is balling yarn. Winding up a hose is in the same league.

We often use different types of rope for winding. The rope is wound onto various spools, usually wooden or cardboard. Remnants of rope can often be bought from hardware stores, spool and all. Wire serves the same purpose and can of course be more time-consuming, as much more wire can fit on a spool.

Another aspect of rope is untying knots. A few minutes of tying simple knots in a length of rope can give an individual a good segment of engaged activity in untying them.

8. Big Colored Clothespins

Big colored clothespins had already become somewhat re-nowned via local Alzheimer newsletters when we received a generous gift from a mysterious visitor. They can be sorted, pinned to the edge of a box or other container, removed from the edge of a box, etc. These have found their way into bushes and low-hanging trees on our grounds. One ap-peared on a bush at the farthest point from our back door; another appeared, gumlike, underneath a picnic table. They can double for more dangerous safety pins and make nifty tie clasps. They could even be used for hanging out clothes. They are available at better hardware stores.

9. Plumbing Supplies (Assorted) (catalogue 4)

Variously sized steel elbows, T's, sleeves, straight lengths, and so on are wonderful to assemble, disassemble, sort, and gen-erally ponder. They are a bit pricey, although less expensive if purchased from a local store than through a specialty cata-logue. (Caution: any metal plumbing item can be used as a very effective projectile. Smaller pieces are more or less bite-sized. These should be left out for independent discovery only with caution.) A base piece, or "root," can be secured to a board for tabletop use, to the side of a workbench, or to some other appropriate surface.

Plastic PVC fixtures can also be very useful. They are also

less expensive. Most PVC fixtures, however, are not threaded; they do not screw apart or together.

10. Nuts and Bolts (catalogs 1, 4, 5, and 12)

A simple board with holes drilled in it provides a task beyond basic sorting and manipulation. This can easily be home made. (The caution for plumbing supplies also applies to nuts and bolts.) Nuts & bolts are also great for sorting.

11. Wooden Shapes

Examples of wooden shapes include "Playful Patterns" (catalog 5) and "Design-a-tile" (catalogs 5, 10, and 12).

12. Wooden Blocks (catalogs 2 and 4)

Many woodworking or furniture factories can supply "odds and ends" (turnings, knobs, caps, etc.) that can be sorted, sanded, painted, etc.

13. Giant Pokeeno Cards

Once upon a time, an activity coordinator in a long-term care fa-cility grew desperate for an acceptable alternative to Beano. She tried Pokeeno; it worked, and it proved to be a popular addition to the activity schedule. Unfortunately, the game cards, as manufactured, were rather small and some players had trouble seeing them. This gave rise to a successful and useful craft project: jumbo-sized playing cards were arranged on large pieces of posterboard, corresponding to the cards in a Pokeeno set, then covered with clear contact paper.

Pokeeno is generally beyond the ability of individuals with dementia. However, the cards have proven very useful. One or more individuals are able to focus for extended peri-ods on the task of matching the cards on the Pokeeno sheets with cards from a deck at hand. This especially appeals to former card players, as it approximates a game of solitaire. This pastime (plus a bottle of nonalcoholic beer) has been a godsend with two very anxious gentlemen, in particular.

• Sorting Tasks •

Sorting is a fairly basic cognitive task. With many folks it is almost automatic: given a pile of colored tiles, many of us will begin to sort them by color. Many of the items listed above as table activities can be sorted.

The arrangements for sorting tasks can vary. Mason jars, which are both transparent and very familiar, make ideal receptacles. So do bowls, candy tins, or simply separated piles. The task can range from selecting a single type of item—"Just the red ones, please"—to sorting out a bowl of items.

Caution needs to be taken with items that might look "good enough to eat." Some very effective sorting items do, in fact, collect the occasional tooth imprint if used over a period of time. With the exception of poker chips, however, I have never seen any "busy-type" items stay long in a resident's mouth; they rarely get beyond the nibbling stage. The ability to discern foreign objects often seems to survive late into the dementia process. Nevertheless, as a rule, items that are even close to bite-sized should never be left around for unsupervised use.

A Baker's Dozen Sorting Tasks

1. Hard Candies
    Hard candies should be of the wrapped variety. They can be purchased fairly cheaply in bulk. A stern caution to be sure that "no one eats any of the candies" provides extra incentive to persevere with the task—and to eat and/or pilfer however many.

    There can be various adaptations of this task. For example, four individuals could each collect a single color. One of the four, of course, could collect a unique assortment without creating any difficulty.

    Caution: This may not be an appropriate pastime for diabetic persons.

2. Odd Socks
    Odd socks are those that have survived after the dryer devoured their mates. An element of success can be introduced by "planting" a number of socks that actually do have mates.

3. Foam Things
    Pieces of a foamlike substance are sold in large plastic containers at most department stores or chain toy stores. They come in various shapes and colors.

4. Pom-poms (as used in crafts)
    Crafts may be beyond the abilities of people with dementia, but pom-poms are not. They are colorful, are fuzzy, and come in

different sizes. One woman used to hoard them under her
mattress as love objects.

5. Colored Pipe Cleaners

6. Cloth Squares/Carpet Samples
   Select various textures, possibly of two or more different sizes.
   There should be a number of each texture and size. Many
   samples of corduroy, wool, and fake fur, for example, would
   be more effective than a bewildering variety of many materials.

7. Artificial Flowers

8. Labeled Envelopes
   Assorted stick-on labels are available at stationery stores and in
   stationery departments. The easiest to sort are the colored
   dots. Those reading "Fragile," "Rush," etc., are more demanding but might also seem more "real."

   Actually attaching the labels to envelopes is a good project
   in itself. Obviously, there is no right or wrong way to this process.

   (A bad idea: an early activity in the A.C.C. program was
   to have participants stuff and/or sort envelopes. This process
   proved a good model for precisely the types of tasks that are
   beyond most individuals with dementia, whether the
   multistage task of folding a piece of paper or the perceptual
   demands of stuffing an envelope.)

9. Baseball Cards (catalog 6)
   Inexpensive facsimiles of classic baseball cards are available. Du-
   plicates would be a good idea.

10. Counting Cubes (or Bears, etc.) (catalog 2)

11. Colored Dominoes (by Fisher Price)
    ("Colored dominoes" was the only task-oriented activity that
    one person would pursue, and she would pursue it for an
    hour at a time, every day, with remarkable attentiveness.)

12. Cups and Saucers
    While a fairly demanding task, sorting out cups and saucers
    can be very engaging for an individual or a team. The task is
    simpler if it involves a matching set, as opposed to mis-
    matched china.

13. Utensils

Always a popular "manipulative," spoons, knives, and forks can be sorted out (and rewashed afterward).

One day, a resident's grandchildren were visiting. They had brought some Lego bricks and started playing on the carpet. Several residents were intrigued, not by the space vehicle being constructed but by the colors of the bricks and the way they fit together.

I started to search for Lego pieces, or similar items that come in basic shapes and are larger than bite size. Some time later, wandering through a large discount store, my gaze was attracted by a display of "bricks." They were plastic, in four basic colors, and about the size of a large brick. They were also on sale for very little money. I bought several packages.

Once I got them home, however, they looked impossibly infantile. I didn't dare actually present them to anyone; they languished in a closet for months. Then, at a staff member's encouragement, I put them out on a table and simply left them. Before long, two women had noticed them and started to work with them, eventually dividing them all by color and then into equal stacks. The plastic bricks continue to be very useful on occasion (and to be found in the most amazing places).

• Games •

Even the most avid game players, whether bridge devotees or Beano addicts, lose their abilities to participate. In a nutshell, the demands of most games fly directly in the face of the disease. The result of attempting most games is more likely to be frustration than enjoyment, a sense of futility rather than achievement. Two games follow, though, that can be effectively used.

Elimination

"Elimination" feels like a card game because it uses playing cards. The only cognitive skill necessary is simple number recognition. As a children's game, it depends on speed, much like "War."

Any number can play, although six is usually about all that can sit around a table. The staff leader deals first, and deals each hand. (The dealer is really a croupier.)

A certain number of cards is dealt to each player. Four is a good number; three cards each makes for a slightly simpler and quicker game. The remaining cards are placed facedown on the table. The dealer reveals the top card. Any player who has that number discards it. If the top card is the eight of clubs, then any eight is eliminated. If a player had all three of the other eights, he or she would discard them all. The first player to get rid of all his or her cards wins! This is a "win/not win" game; no one actually loses. Individuals often become empty-handed at the same time.

Hands may be played close to the chest or wide open in this game. Secrecy does not matter (unless it seems important to individual players).

An explanation may be offered that we'll "start off slow, then speed up as we go along." Then we simply play at a pace appropriate to the group.

Three-in-a-Row

Beano may be an inevitable fact of geriatric life in the United States, if only because it is such a familiar and enjoyable pastime for so many. However, to mix Beano with dementia often results in near cruelty. Some long-term care settings provide their participants with helpers when it's time for the cognitively impossible Beano challenge. It is hard to imagine a more futile, dependent, or passive occupation. In fact, few individuals with dementia would be engaged by—or sit still for—such activity.

Three-in-a-Row resembles Beano but is significantly more appropriate to a range of abilities with dementia. Generally, about a third of the A.C.C. residents and most adult day program participants have been able to play this game either independently or with minimal assistance. Like Beano/Bingo, it is a lotto-type game, but it requires only simple number recognition.

A Three-in-a-Row "card" is made from an 8½" × 11" sheet of paper. (The sheet could be laminated, but some individuals do enjoy writing on them.) It looks similar to a Bingo card, but with only nine squares. There is a number in each square. The left squares contain randomly selected numbers between 1 and 9; the center squares, numbers between 10 and 19; and the right squares, numbers between 20 and 29.

The columns can be color coded (say, green, red, and blue) to provide additional cuing. It's that simple, but it feels like a "real" game.

Fifty-two Pick-up (a game of diversion)

At least half-seriously, as a distraction from anxiety, even as an intervention for agitation, "Fifty-two Pick-up" can be effective. The task of helping, that is, picking up the cards (or whatever else) that you have just dropped, will often override whatever anxiety an individual may be feeling. If you happen to drop a pile of color-coded envelopes, the individual might further be willing to help you sort them (perhaps grumbling about it, to start). Sometimes the pure shock of your dropping a pile of whatever will divert an individual's focus from, for example, "getting out, to find my car!"

On one occasion, Olga was highly agitated, bent on throwing everyone "out of her house." A staff member dropped a pile of envelopes and magazines in front of her. Olga was certainly not motivated to assist in picking them up, but her attention shifted to making sure the items were picked up properly. This provided enough diversion to begin the process of redirecting her energies. On another occasion, a cup of coffee spilled on the kitchen floor provided a similar diversion.

• Social Activities •

One universally noted aspect of dementia is the preservation of manners. It is an amazing phenomenon to see folks rise to the social occasion. Social activities provide opportunities for these manners, or social graces, to continue being used. Social gatherings are also—not incidentally—very reassuring; it feels secure to be there.

At A.C.C. we tend to use these activities in the late afternoon, the traditional teatime. A major aspect of such events is socializing the interaction (verbal and nonverbal) around a table. Once triggered, possibly by a staff member or volunteer, this sort of cheerful social intercourse tends to keep itself going.

The fact that social events typically involve food is not accidental. We have found—during, for example, post-holiday crusades to cut down on snacks—that a little something in the late afternoon helps limit "sundown" anxiety. Put a different way, hunger is highly agitating. After all, a snack in the late afternoon, to tide us over, is normal for most of us. The benefits of providing nourishment and hydration are especially relevant with dementia.

Another aspect of such activities is that they can involve a majority of residents and are relatively easy to conduct: a staff member and a volunteer can generally manage just fine. They can also be planned to require minimal preparation and cleanup.

Typical examples of social activities include the ubiquitous tea (hot or, in season, iced), ice cream socials (from dish or cone to sundaes or floats), any beverage with cookies or something more healthful, and watermelon. (Watermelon is ideal food for the purpose, given its ease of preparation, its color, sweet taste, lack of dietary contraindications, ease of eating with fork or with fingers, and the essential, time-consuming task of removing the seeds. Watermelon seeds are familiar to most folks, unlike, for instance, those terrifying tiny "bugs" in kiwi fruit.)

Any of the above can be combined with an entertainment—before, during, or after. The only provisos are that offering a choice sometimes creates enough talk to be distracting during, say, a musical program, and teacups and saucers rattle a lot.

A "High tea," for example, can involve almost unlimited chores, including washing and setting the tables, folding napkins, preparing food, sorting cups and saucers, filling the sugar bowl (especially task-orienting if done with sugar packets), host/hostessing, and serving.

·: 5 :·

Exercise

When people think of dementia, they often picture folks engaged in the exercise of walking. The abilities of folks with dementia to walk steadily, independently, and for long distances are legendary. The media frequently focus on physical activity when reporting on Adult Day Programs and special dementia-care units in long-term care facilities. Exercise, ranging from a basic sitting-down group routine to adapted sports such as volleyball, not only is active and visible but also contradicts many negative stereotypes of dementia and of aging in general.

In designing the activity program at the A.C.C., we recognized that structured physical exercise would be a vital component of each day. Much of the available literature recommended exercise, if only simple walking, as a primary tool in releasing energy, maintaining physical fitness promoting a sense of well-being and accomplishment, and managing agitation. Experience and common sense suggested that people generally feel better, are more relaxed, and are more cognitively functional after exercise. Many traditional reality-orientation classes began with some basic exercise for this reason. The difference in an individual's involvement and ability was obvious.

Our first exercise group began with a known quantity: a basic, sitdown routine. The routine rapidly evolved, guided by the folks' abilities and energy (both of which were abundant).

We did not use any prerecorded exercise tape. In the first place, few if any dementia-specific tapes were available at that time. Moreover, any recorded routine tends to limit spontaneity; it may be necessary to alter the rhythm or count of a specific movement, to suit the participants. It can also be difficult, following a formatted routine, to incorporate the unique contributions of group participants. Above all, a "set" routine could stifle the spontaneous humor often present in an exercise group for people with dementia.

The chairs were gone by the third day. There seemed to be no limit to what the folks could–and wanted to—do.

On the fourth day, we found the limit.

The group was conducted in our living room—a fairly large, carpeted area. The next logical progression in our routine was to floor exercises. At that, several women balked: they were not about to get down on the floor wearing dresses and nylons. Moreover, at least two of the women were not, by long personal preference, likely candidates for any kind of slacks, let alone sweatsuits!

Having found the general parameters, we rapidly developed our own exercise routine. It includes many aspects of standard routines, both geriatric and otherwise. The actual routine and the movements in it never stopped evolving. Many adaptations and variations, based on individuals' special needs and challenges, crept in. Spontaneous movements, including individuals' approximations of a given move, were often the best inspirations.

We used an exercise tape (of music only) for each session. These tapes were specially designed and made, each following a format: beginning with a sequence of very relaxing music, gradually building to a peak, then slowing down again. Each tape was thirty minutes long, the approximate duration of each session. The tapes were played on a portable cassette player so the group leader(s) could have some control over the timing of the tape. The flip side of each tape began at a moderate energy level, progressing to quieter rhythms. These were designed for use after the actual exercise routine.

Each tape consisted of music from one decade. The idea was to use one tape per day, every week, as a mnemonic aid. Thus, Monday was music from the 1920s, Tuesday from the 1930s, and so on; Saturday was intended to be more or less the present. Not surprisingly, the most effective tape was the 1940s; we still use it for a variety of up-tempo rhythmic activities. The least effective was the 1960s tape (although it tended to be popular with the staff). The "present" tape self-destructed almost as soon as it was played, probably as an act of mercy by the dementia guardian angel. We rapidly learned, in any event, that residents relished a rest come Saturday morning. (See Chapter 1.)

• Stand-up Routine •

Preparation

Furniture is rearranged to afford as much room as possible while minimizing commotion (initially and after the group). The stand-up routine is conducted in our living-room area.

Participants are encouraged to join the circle with positive, cheerful, matter-of-fact invitations, such as "It's time for our morning exercises; please join us" or "We're all getting together; we don't want to start without you." Often a smile, a beckon of the head and/or hand is sufficient encouragement.

Gathering in a circle, with everyone holding hands, helps keep the group reasonably intact and provides a sense of togetherness. It also helps the participants to keep their balance—a safety concern for many individuals. Holding hands is a reassuring activity; hands full of hands feel great. There is also bound to be at least one individual whose hands need warming up! Once bonded, the circle will tend to stay together during the individual, or separated, sequence.

Routine

The group should be encouraged: "Everybody's different; do what feels comfortable for you." All exercises should be done to tolerance.

Introduce and slowly demonstrate all movements. There should be one or more practice movements. Repeat each movement at least three times, then in increments of three (six, nine, twelve, etc.). Individuals are not physically assisted to perform any specific movement, to do it "right," or to do it at all. Most direct help feels demeaning. Eye contact, expecially with eyebrows raised in encouragement, is far more effective.

The basic sequence of movement is a gradual progression from head to toe. Generally, left and right are not important; many individuals not afflicted with dementia are challenged by such lateral awareness.

Whether one moves the right or left arm correctly is usually unimportant; to assist someone with the correct side, or to move at all, is a clear indication that he or she has failed. This is not physical therapy. In terms of bodily awareness, one side as opposed to the other is significant. Of course, a problem might arise if an individual did all the movements with, say, only the right leg. Directions—the "count"—should stress "one side, the other side," rather than "left, right, left, right."

I. Warm-up
   A. Breathing
      Emphasize deep breathing throughout the routine: "Please take a good, deep, breath. Breathe in through your nose, out through your mouth. In with the good air, out with the bad. (And don't forget to let it out!)"
   B. Head and Neck
      "These are relaxing exercises. Be sure to stand up straight."
      1. Up and down: a slowly nodding, exaggerated "yes" motion. Cue: "Look straight ahead, then down at your toes, then straight ahead again."
      2. Side to side. Cue: "Turn your head to one side, then the other, like looking over your shoulder."
      3. Tilt: tilt head to right, then left; alternate. Cue: "As if you're trying to touch your right ear to your right shoulder."
   C. Shoulders
      1. Shrugs, up and down.
      2. Shrugs, right shoulder.
      3. Shrugs, left shoulder.
      4. Shrugs, right, then left, alternating.
   D. Torso Tilting
      Cue: Tilt to the left, then right; alternate.
   E. Torso Bending
      Arms up, bend back, bend arms with eyes focused on the person across the circle. Cue: "Slowly bend over forward; keep your eyes up." Caution: "Keep your eyes up as you bend over. Keep your eyes on the person across from you."

F. Swing and Sway (hips)
   1. Shimmy: Thrust hips to right, then left; alternate.
   2. Twist (like the dance).

II. Free-standing Routine
(Break the group with either "You're doing great! Give yourself a hand," or "Pat your thighs.")

A. Shoulders
   1. Bear hug. Cue: "Give yourself a good big hug, like you mean it."
   2. Rock-a-bye baby: Exactly that.

B. Arms
   1. The "one-two." Cue: "Arms up; make a fist. Now, with your left hand, reach out; then right, continue. Like boxing."
   2. "Accuse." The leader stands in the center. Cue: "Please accuse me: point at me with your right hand!"
      - ("What did I do?")
      - Now touch your nose.
      - Point with your left hand.
      - Now touch your nose.
      - Now repeat, both hands at once.
   3. Scratch your ear. Cue: "Stretch your left hand over your head, as if you want to scratch your right ear."
      - Repeat, right hand to left ear.
      - Alternate.
   4. Swimming. Various strokes, one or more: crawl, dog-paddle, back stroke, tread water.
   5. Ceiling poke: Reach up, "Touch the ceiling." Then slouch, relax. Repeat.
   6. "Physical culture." Hands on shoulders: Reach up with both hands; return hands to shoulders.
      - Reach up with the right hand only.
      - Reach up with the left hand only.
      - Alternate.
   7. "Falling leaves/Hallelujah." Reach up, shake hands, let hands fall, then raise them up again, repeat.

III.   Legs

   A.   Cue: "Join hands again." Note: With some of the following, individuals confusing their left and right can be a problem. If you and I are holding hands and I am on your right, if you kick your right leg to your right and I kick my left leg to the left, we may kick each other, fall, or become generally discombobulated.

   1.   Side step (two-step). Step to the right, then left;

   2.   Leg shakes. Cue: "Give your left leg a shake; stop. Shake; stop."
      • Repeat with the right leg.

   3.   Knee lifts. Left leg: stretch, lift up, then down.
      • Repeat with the right leg.
      • Option: Left, then right; repeat (marching in place).

   4.   Knee thrusts. Slowly lift the left knee, stick out the left foot, and down.
      • Repeat with the right knee.
      • Option: Alternate knees (can-can).

   5.   Leg circles. Stick the left leg out, make three quick circles, then stop.
      • Repeat with the right leg.

   6.   Kicks. Standing stationary: simple kicks with the left leg.
      • Kick with the right leg.
      • Alternate legs (cakewalk).

   B.   Dance (Optional)

   1.   The Hat Dance. Felt/straw hats are placed in the center. In rhythm, the circle dances in, touches or stomps on the hats, then dances back; repeat, in and out.

   2.   Follow the Leader/Round Robin Dancing. The leader starts a slow motion; everybody follows. The next person in line adds any movement, which the group then follows, or mirrors. The added movement may be something more or less unintentional: a shrug ("I don't know"), a smile, a frown, etc. One day, a participant stuck out her tongue at the group leader. She was smiling, and everyone else smiled and greatly en-

joyed following her lead. It was so much fun that I in-
corporated it into the next day's routine.

3. Parachute. A parachute can be used at various junc-
tures in the routine, though only once per session.
(Parachutes are available from many sources, such as
catalogs 8, 10, 12, and 13.) (Note: Those designed for
children are lighter and more appropriate for indoor
use.)

IV. Cool Down
Emphasize rhythmic breathing. Some gentle swaying, side-to-
side, usually fits this section. Various visualizations can be used
as well, although only to a limited degree: it's tricky to visualize
yourself in a spring field of dandelions if you have limited attentiveness and recall.

There will be individuals who are unable to join in this standing routine but will participate while sitting. They form a second, more or less separate, group. Extra chairs should be provided for others who may drop out during the routine. At
times, there might even be as many participants sitting as standing.

Some may be altogether unable to participate. A separate
group, usually gathered around a table, is required. This
group's activities are sometimes as basic as rolling Nerf balls or
punch balls back and forth.

One gentleman simply loathed any and all exercise groups
and would loudly ridicule such activities. He did well, though,
enjoying an additional glass of cranberry juice, seated at a table,
facing out a window toward the garden, often with a magazine
of choice, often with a companion. As he had a profound hearing loss, Vernon was unaware of the groups in progress: "out of
sight, out of mind."

Problems

We perceived three major difficulties with the stand-up exercise routine. First, it was staff-intensive, requiring at least three members or
volunteers: one for the stand-up group, one for the table group, and
one to "float."

Second, the stand-up group made certain demands on individual
staff members. For one thing, it required special voice-control tech-

niques, and staff members who had naturally soft and/or high-pitched voices had an uphill struggle with this format. Staff members who were of particularly short stature also had difficulty conducting the group. Others had difficulty with the physical demands that the group made. Further, although all efforts were made to limit the commotion created by moving furniture and gathering a group, the process still created a high level of energy.

Finally, group-leader burn-out tended to set in quickly, suddenly, and hard. Largely as a change for the group leaders, we shifted to a sit-down routine. This rapidly became our standard exercise format.

• Sit-Down Routine •

We hold this group in our dining room area, where it happens to be inconvenient to control the tape player. Before long, there was a consensus that *not* using the tapes made for less general hubbub. For example, individuals coming to breakfast during the exercise sessions were more likely to be comfortable eating in the dining room, even joining in with some movements, as opposed to fleeing to the much more tranquil kitchen or other areas.

It appeared that the tapes had little effect on folks' rhythmic participation; the beat of a given exercise was set and maintained primarily by the group leader. (Granted, some group leaders did benefit somewhat by having the tapes to guide them.) The tapes also raised the room's energy level and agitated some individuals not engaged in one of the exercise groups.

Again, adaptations for dementia began to appear. Our new adult day program director had previously been a trainer for a local manufacturing company and had conducted exercise classes emphasizing fine-motor acuity and eye-hand coordination. Some of these simple movements proved ideal for our purposes.

Preparation

The tables are moved, as slightly, slowly, and quietly as possible, to create a large enough space in the center of the room. The chairs are then turned, spaced a comfortable distance apart, to create a circle. (At one point we tried an arrangement in which the chairs were staggered.

This created more space for each individual to move his or her arms during the routine, while retaining a circular seating arrangement. It created a larger problem, though, which led to its abandonment: lack of eye contact and sight lines with the leader.)

Routine

I.   Smile and Sing
The leader greets the participants, as individually as possible. It is important to establish focus and attentiveness, using whatever it takes. Brief reality-orientation discussions (date, day, etc.), weather, tall tales, jokes, and old songs are all commonly used. Frequent songs include *Down by the Old Mill Stream, Let Me Call You Sweetheart, Oh, How I Hate to Get Up in the Morning, Oh, What a Beautiful Morning, Good Morning to You!* (more or less as a joke), and, on a rainy day, *Rain, Rain, Go Away.*

II. Head and Shoulders

   A.   Introduction
   Remind all participants to sit back in their chairs with their feet flat on the floor.

   B.   Breathing
   Any number of basic breathing, relaxation techniques can be used. Verbal cues/closure phrases can be included: "Let's start with a good, deep, breath. In with the good air, out with the bad. In with the new air, out with the old. In with the fresh air, out with the stale." These cues (and many others) can be repeated throughout the routine.
      Breathing exercises can be followed by another exercise, often very difficult for people to do in the morning: a smile! (The exercise can be to "Smile (big!), then stop," or "Smile, then frown!")
      A note about counting: Counting along to a given movement is often a good idea, and it may develop spontaneously. In fact, many participants often expect to count, in cadence, and will initiate it. Most people join in more or less automatically, as if the counting fosters a sense of social security, of belonging. A rhythmic count gives the leader an ideal tool with which to maintain an even pace.

As with singing some individuals will tend to speed up (see Chapter 6). Again, as with singing, it is vital that the leader—in a gentle, subtle, but definite, way—retain control over the proceedings. This is especially important when there are participants who are counting on the off-beat or who exuberantly and immediately say the number to follow (that is, to say, "6" as soon as they hear the count of "5"). If people get flustered, they tend to stop. On the other hand, rushing the pace, while exercising, could actually be physically dangerous. To retain control of the cadence, it is helpful to insert the word *and* between each count, and accent the terminal *d:* "One an*d* two an*d* three," and so on.

The number of repetitions of each exercise may vary from day to day. If the participants are largely the same from Monday through Friday, then the number of reps may increase through the week. Even if the number of reps does not vary from day to day, there can still be a handy excuse for adding calendar reminders: "Since it's Wednesday, let's do twelve of these." (Rarely will anyone comment, "But don't we always do twelve, regardless of what day it is?")

During movements that alternate from left to right, it may be helpful for the leader to count "left and right and left and right," rather than a numerical count. Again, the count is for guidance, or cuing, not for mastery of which side is which. Verbal cues can include, "What's good for the left side is good for the right." A more specific cue could be, "What's good for the left shoulder is good for the right." This cue can be repeated throughout the routine, focusing on the different body parts being exercised.

C. Wake-up
Yawn and stretch, free form. (Noise with the yawning is optional.)
Cue: "What do people do when they first wake up in the morning?"

D. Nodding
Touch the chin to the chest, then look straight ahead; repeat.

Caution: The head should not "nod" back.)

E. Head Twist
Cue: "This is a 'city' exercise: look over your shoulder to see who's behind you!"

1. Look over the left shoulder.
2. Look over the right shoulder.
3. Turn head left, then right (like an exaggerated "No").

F. Shoulder Shrugs
Cue: "As if you just heard the dumbest question you've ever heard in your life: 'I dunno.'"

1. Up and down, to the count
2. Left, to the count
3. Right, to the count
4. Alternating: left, then right; one, then the other.

G. Ceiling Scratch
Cue: "Reach up with both hands and touch the ceiling. (Be careful of the ceiling fan.)" Stretch, then relax; repeat.
Options:

1. Try inhaling when reaching up, exhaling while lowering the arms ("Like an old-fashioned bellows").
2. Raise hands, then shake: "Hallelujah!"
3. Raise the left hand; repeat.
4. Raise the right hand; repeat.
5. Alternate.

Caution: As a rule, exercises in which the arms rise above the shoulder should not follow one another.

H. Hug Yourself
Cue: "Give yourself a big hug, like you mean it." Hug, open (arms stretching out); repeat.

I. *Rock-a-bye Baby*
Make the movements with the song. (A discussion of the implications of this lullaby's odd lyrics is optional. The lyrics definitely underscore the importance of the message as opposed to the actual words!)

III. Arms and Hands
    A. "Physical Culture" Arm Lifts
        Hands on shoulders; raise hands, then back to shoulders.
        1. Raise both hands, replace, to the count.
        2. Raise the left hand, replace, to the count.
        3. Raise the right hand, replace, to the count.
        4. Raise the left, then the right, etc., to the count.
    B. Shoulder Touches
        1. Arms out, palms up, bend the left elbow, touch fingers to the left shoulder.
        2. Right elbow.
        3. Both at once.
        4. Left hand to the right shoulder
        5. Right hand to the left shoulder
    C. Ear Touches ("Reach Over")
        Cue: "As if you wanted to scratch your ears."
        1. With the left hand, reach over head, touch the right ear, then back. Repeat, to the count.
        2. With right ear, the same, to the count.
        3. Alternate, saying, "left, then right," etc.
    D. "One-Two"
        Caution: Be sure to do this facing front! Cue: "Like boxing: raise your arms, make fists, then 'one, two; one, two.'"
    E. Open and Close
        Arms relaxed: make a fist (both hands), then open; close, open, etc.
        Options:
        1. Follow the leader. The leader varies the cadence; the group tries to follow directions.
        2. Same: left, then right; left, right; right, right; left, left; etc.
    F. Butterfly
        Cue: "Put your hands together as if you're praying."
        1. Hands open, fingers apart, heels of the hands remaining together.

2. Hands open, fingers together, heels of the hands separating.
3. Bend wrists to the left, then right.
Note: Hand exercises tend to suggest *He's Got the Whole World in His Hands.*

G. Rowing
Cue: "How many have ever rowed a boat? Let's do it. Lean forward, grab those oars, and pull." (The song, obviously, is *Row, Row, Row Your Boat*.)

H. Scissors
Arms up; simply cross, then straight; cross, etc.

I. Chopping Wood
Clearly a movement ripe with reminiscence. Hands are clasped together and held above the head, as if raising an ax, then "chop!" The count works best on the "chop," the "ax" raised on "and." Other "chores" can include churning butter (using one of several styles of churn), a two-person cross-cut saw, shoveling, turning an old wringer, etc. We often pause at this point for a work-oriented song, such as *I've Been Working on the Railroad.*

IV. Legs and Feet
This might begin with a slow "walk": simply moving the feet, "waking them up."

A. Toe Lifts (to the count)

B. Lift Heels (to the count)

C. Leg Lifts/Kicks
Cuing can include encouragement to "touch the ceiling with your toes—just be careful of the fan."
1. First stretch left, then right.
2. Kicks with the left leg, to the count.
3. Kicks with the right leg, to the count.
4. Kicks, alternating.
5. While sitting, lift both legs (and quickly let them down to the floor).

D. Cross Legs (at the knees)
Move toes in circles, then switch; fidget (like "waiting in a doctor's office"), switch again, etc.

E. Leg Circles

    1. Lift the left leg, make three circles, then drop the leg to the floor. Repeat, with circles in the opposite direction.

    2. Repeat with the right (the "other") leg.

F. Knee Lifts

    1. Stretch left, then right.

    2. Lift the left knee, to the count.

    3. Lift the right knee, to the count.

    4. Alternate, left, then right. This turns into a marching movement; just add *Over There,* or *Tipperary* and march!

V. Punch Balls/Bombardment! (or Parachute)

Note: Punch balls "fly," whereas balloons "float." Other balls—even nerf balls or beach balls—can hit too hard and be traumatizing, although the effects of the trauma may not appear for as long as a half-hour after the event. Even punch balls (for example, striking a participant by surprise in the glasses) can be shocking enough to require some good-natured TLC.

VI. Accessories

Many exercise routines employ props, ranging from batons to scarves to bottles (full or empty). Different types of elastic (such as waistband elastic) can be useful, both in individual lengths and in lengths long enough to surround, and be used by, the group as a whole.

A group of participants with dementia is always a potentially volatile situation. Tempers can flare in an instant; with typical lack of impulse control, the friendly tap or cuff can become a full-force blow. Although wooden dowels are frequently used in various exercise routines, an accidental hit from a wooden rod is likely to hurt and will probably feel like an assault. I prefer to avoid such potential weaponry.

We sometimes use a collection of yarn cones, or spindles, as used in fabric mills, for the same purposes. These are like the hand cones used in occupational and physical therapy. Ours happen to be plastic, open at both ends, and up to a foot long. Held between the hands, these add a unique aspect to a routine. They are particularly good in mimicking work motions, such as turning a crank, sawing with a two-person crosscut saw, churning butter, etc.

These cones add another aspect as well. They are stored in a small (13 gal.) round plastic trash barrel. Participants usually start manipulating them as soon as they take them out of the barrel, using them as trumpets, antlers, kazoos, etc. Individuals are particularly intrigued by the way things look when seen through a "telescope" and by the sound heard through an "ear trumpet."

For the conclusion, the barrel is placed in the middle, and the cones are returned—airborne. Most folks can be persuaded to try their luck; those who get the cone into the box can get another shot, and so on, as desired.

VII. *The Hokey Pokey*

Both the song and the routine of *Hokey Pokey* are old enough to be familiar and even automatic. The routine can easily be adapted for either sitting or standing. As with the stand-up routine, it is helpful for standing individuals to hold hands. We generally use this as a standing routine. It is helpful to have the group first stamp their feet a while, then stand either to a count of "one, two, three!" or to *God Bless America* (see Chapter 6). So, instead of, "You do the *Hokey Pokey* and you turn yourself about," the leader can simply direct a slight knee-bend, stepping side to side, or "twist your hips about," and *"that's* what it's all about." A good beginning "to get the feel of it" is to sway a bit: slowly sway to the left, then (slowly) to the right. This often triggers the slogan, "Swing and sway with   [Sammy Kaye!]." The sway can become a swing, accompanied by *Swing Low, Sweet Chariot*. Different movements during the dance can include the head, shoulders, stomach, hands, hips. It's hard to do, say, the left hand and then the right hand; your left hand will be holding my right, and so on. However, everyone's legs can be moved separately, usually to a slower pace. It's possible to put "your whole self" in, out, and shake it all about, too, at an even slower pace.

VIII. Cool Down, Deep Breathing, etc. (same as the Free-standing Routine)

Pros and Cons

There are trade-offs between the standing and sitting formats. The sit-down group is less demanding for staff leaders: as participants are seated, their attention is more easily sustained; group cohesion is more easily maintained (folks are less likely to wander off or need to sit down); once established, the group can easily be conducted by one person, with someone else floating or keeping an eye out. Moreover, the fact that virtually everyone is physically able to join the main group is a bonus. Without the structure of a tape, there tends to be more spontaneous singing, joking, and storytelling. There is also more flexibility in the routine, to lengthen one movement, shorten another, or repeat a third.

On the other hand, while the stand-up group could provide fairly significant aerobic exercise, little if any of the sitting routine goes beyond the level of active range of motion.

The two routines, sit-down and stand-up, can naturally be combined. A standing sequence at the end of a sitting routine can be a boon; too much sitting is too much. Some leg exercises, such as marching, feel more natural when standing. Others, such as pushing up on toes, are much more effective. Still others, of course, such as crossing the knees or raising both legs at the same time, can't really be done (safely) when standing!

• Walking •

Walking is the easiest, most natural, and possibly the most beneficial exercise of all.

We are fortunate that the A.C.C. is located in a quiet residential neighborhood, largely surrounded by woods. The hills we need to contend with are gradual and—with the notable exception of our own driveway—quite minor.

The sidewalks in the neighborhood have proven to be a mixed blessing. They tend to help walkers keep together, going in the same direction, and they tend to be dry and, in winter, plowed. Unfortunately, some places are cracked and uneven. More dangerous, there are stretches where the sides are steep (some places a matter of inches, some places more than a foot). With the perceptual deficits normal for dementia, folks tend not to perceive the drop-offs. Having seen several folks trip and plummet to the pavement off the edge of sidewalks, we generally avoid them.

Our group hikes rapidly became familiar in the neighborhood. Certain routes are better than others by virtue of shade or traffic at a given time of day. We gauge distances by designated landmarks.

In the past two years, we have had access to a nearly ideal walking opportunity: an 1100-acre family estate. A well-maintained gravel road, extending from the end of our road, runs through lush hay fields, woods, and meadows. This resource has been astonishing. Staff members have been known to feel guilty for having such an enjoyable experience on "company time."

There are a few ground rules for our hikes.

1. We avoid the middle to late afternoon hours, when there is a surge in traffic, largely school-related. Even the short stretch of street we have to travel to get to the estate can be problematical: there is one tricky intersection and we have to use the sidewalk during those hours.

2. "Expect the unexpected" is a crucial byword with any outing. Generally, no individual helper walks with more than one resident. Two helpers, however, can usually handle a group of six fairly reliable folks. With groups larger than six or if the six include individuals of very differing abilities, then there is likely to be a minority who need to turn back. Obviously, someone needs to accompany them.

3. We generally adhere to a helper-to-resident ratio of 1:3. Thus, a hiking party of twelve residents might require four helpers: two to turn back with, say, five folks, and two to continue with the rest. The walkers who will turn back can often be anticipated. More than once, however, our expectations (and times of return) have been quite mistaken! Exceeding the ratio is risky.

4. We always have a "caboose"—one helper in the rear of the procession, behind everyone else. No resident gets behind the caboose.

5. A helper should be at dangerous corners. A person with dementia will tend to walk in a straight line unless he or she meets an obstacle. For example, if the route of a walk turns at a certain intersection (no matter how small and quiet), then a

helper should be positioned to block folks from walking straight into the intersection. If a group is walking along a dock, to climb into a boat, then someone should stand at the end of the dock. A straight line would lead many individuals with dementia directly into the water!

6. It is usually better for helpers *not* to hold hands with folks; it slows them down. While speed is not important as such, the more spread-out a group, the trickier the helpers' task. All too often, the act of offering to hold an individual's hand presumes that assistance is required. Most often, it is not. However, residents tend to seek out another resident who will walk at a pace similar to their own.

It may be a good idea for the caboose to hold hands, if only to prevent an individual or two from lagging even further behind.

Two people holding hands are obviously going to be walking side by side. This can be a danger in a road. One helper holding hands with two folks creates a line of three, side by side, which can be less than safe. As with riding bicycles, the safest walking formation is more or less single file.

Walking is rarely all that happens during a walk. Hikes tend to be very social times as well. Smiles abound; there is a lot of joking, singing, laughter. There is also—quite naturally—a good deal of stimulation for all five senses.

Outdoor walks, especially, can provide wonderful chances for a wide range of specific, goal-oriented cognitive therapy techniques. These might include:

- Object naming: "Look at that blue (sky)"; "What would you call that bird? (A pigeon?)"
- Discrimination: "Would you call that a car or a truck?" "What kind of tree would you say that was?"
- Reminiscing: "Do you like dandelion greens?" "Did you ever ride to school on a bus?" "Did your kids ride bicycles like that?"
- Recall stimulation: "Who squashed that caterpillar a while ago?" "Isn't this where we saw the deer yesterday? Now which way do we turn to get back?"

- Closure exercises: "That's not far—just a hop, skip, and a . . ." "Make hay while . . ." "Oh, what a beautiful . . ." "Blue skies, smiling at me! Nothing but blue skies . . ."

A Bad Idea

Early on, exploring the neighborhood and having a vision of the ideal walking environment, we had a brainstorm.

At the end of one very quiet, dead-end residential street is a large, even quieter cemetery. Further, the cemetery also provided a perfect connector from the end of one dead-end street to another.

When we got into the cemetery, once everyone had time to realize where we were, a very peculiar reaction—part panic, part fear—set in. We turned around at once, diverted attention to the clouds, a dog in a yard, or something, barely averting a truly catastrophic reaction.

We have avoided cemeteries, however tranquil, ever since.

Indoor Walks

The A.C.C. is designed to provide an indoor track. Twenty times around is roughly equivalent to a mile. The track, however, consists of the regular corridors. Some adaptations are required to make the track self-cuing. Among these are strategically hung signs that read:

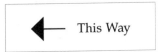

This track has many distractions, especially chances to go straight ahead. Some preparation is necessary: closing doors (except those through which we need to walk), turning off the television, arranging "baffles" such as chairs or sofas kitty-cornered near doorways. It is helpful to close blinds and curtains: sight-seers tend to stop.

Our administrator's office is at the end of one long hall: the end of a logical beeline. Many residents are accustomed to visiting in there to begin with. During walks, we place an old dressing screen at an angle hiding the door (out of sight, out of mind) and the "This Way" sign on the screen helps to guide the procession.

It is important that everyone walk, as much as possible, in the same direction. This definitely includes staff, visitors, bewildered tradespersons, and so on. When encountering individuals going in the opposite direction, many folks tend to stop and turn around.

We have had falls during our walks, though relatively few and with relatively little injury. Invariably, however, folks have fallen because they lost their balance, and they lost their balance because someone in front of them stopped.

Bottlenecks do occur, and they can be both annoying and dangerous. Most folks, though, can generally go at their own pace, passing slower folks. (In our situation, this has always been counterclockwise. It simply seemed the direction of fewer distractions, though there isn't really much to choose from. Individuals who are in a "contrary" mood, today or in general, often make a point of walking "against the grain." Some walk "opposite" on a given day; some never choose to walk in the same direction as the crowd.) A helper at a corner, using typical, exaggerated traffic cop gestures, is sometimes useful.

Once the march is established, the momentum tends to sustain itself. Staff vigilance is essential to assist individuals who are walking at much faster or much slower speeds, as well as to redirect those who have become turned around. Naturally, as folks progress in their disease, they grow more easily distracted. Some require near-constant one-to-one support to keep going, let alone to continue in the "correct" direction.

Indoors as well as out, a team of two, at minimum, is essential to ensure the safety of all walkers. Additional helpers can increase overall socialization: singing, chatting, and so on. They can also concentrate on noninvolved individuals, providing motivational help to those who need extra encouragement or a partner, or alternative activity—perhaps sitting in a quiet, sunny spot, reading a magazine. Additional staff members or volunteers (sometimes including residents and A.D.P participants) can also provide guarded assistance to those with limited mobility and/or endurance.

These walks are very social times. Some folks have a near-automatic "cheer-up and smile" reaction to the simple act of walking, and especially walking with a partner or partners. There is a lot more than walking going on: noticing how much warmer the sun is as we walk through it; noticing the picture of the collie mother and puppy on the wall every time by; noting how much the base of the old dressing screen resembles a nest of snakes; noticing the cats lolling in the sun.

Folks "peter out" at their own pace. The length of a given walk can be quite unpredictable. Walks tend to wind down gradually rather than stopping suddenly. The more consistently the walks occur, as in winter, the longer they tend to last.

Walks seem ideally suited, indoors and out, for late morning—a perfect lead-in to lunch. However, we find that midafternoon walks generally do not—if adequately supervised—create any undue agitation, although they tend to last for a shorter time.

We usually use a "marching tape" to walk to. Music lends a strong cue for walking. *The Stars and Stripes Forever* tends to trigger a marching response. Variety, however, is important; no two marches should be played back-to-back. Milder tempos are preferable: *The Blue Danube* and *The Tennessee Waltz*. Singing while walking is also a common urge. Selected sing-along numbers are included in each tape.

A Bad Idea

In originally designing the A.C.C. program, we tried to keep several hallmark behaviors in mind. Among these were "sundowning" and sleep disturbances (micro-arousal). If exercise releases anxiety and promotes relaxation, we reasoned, then it would be logical to include an exercise period in the early evening. An evening "march" seemed to offer a social and fairly easily conducted after-supper program that should work.

We made an evening marching tape that started very quietly and progressed through waltzes to Sousa marches. The flip side of this tape consisted of "evening calm-down music," starting with a fairly quiet selection (*Blue Shadows on the Trail*) and progressing to the downright soporific (*Beautiful Dreamer*). This was to accompany a "quiet social" after the marches, presumably with snacks prepared by staff members and nonstrolling residents. Appropriate beverages were to be offered, including hot milk, chamomile tea, and cocktails of choice.

The march idea fizzled. Many folks enjoyed the marching; they simply kept marching more or less all night! Others found the level of activity (and the volume of the tapes) disturbing. We were clearly helping folks march into sensory overload, exhaustion, and anything but relaxation.

Those original marching tapes turned out to be too frenetic: too much Sousa. The "quiet" tapes, however, were fairly effective: relaxing and, to some extent, orienting. But there was a special problem with one of the calm-down tapes. The agitating song was *Tonight,* from *West Side Story.* The problem was not the song—a good idea in itself—but the rendition: it was sung, beautifully, by Anna Maria Alberghetti. The ear with dementia does not appreciate the coloratura!

∴ 6 ∴

Music

Music can be magical. Of all the therapies, music offers the best hope of providing a generally effective set of approaches, techniques, and tools for people with dementia. There is a power in music that can transcend language. Musical memories often outlast verbal abilities. What appear to be long-lasting verbal memories—nursery rhymes, for example—owe more to the music in the language than to the words themselves.

Music can be calming and motivating, can wake us up and wind us down, can stir up pleasant memories, and can provide many moments for folks to shine. Music can also be a uniquely agitating, infuriating, traumatizing aspect of one's work, day-to-day or minute-to-minute.

As Joan Butterfield Whitcomb suggested in her excellent piece, "Thanks for the Memory," "Interaction with an Alzheimer's patient through music . . . is communicating with the healthy aspects of the whole person . . . Deep understanding and a sense of well-being are restored for a precious interval of time. The memory of the interaction soon fades from the patient's mind, but the positive affect elicited by it remains and can be built upon by other therapeutic interactions" (Whitcomb, 1989, p. 22).

Most people feel inadequate as musicians or singers. Most health-care workers feel inadequate as music therapists or even sing-along leaders, yet most dementia caregivers use music in therapy, diversion, and motivation every day. Granted, it's tricky to lead an a cappella sing-along if you're tone deaf or can't carry a tune in a basket. It's also tough to sing along with a piano player if you've never heard the tune before. Most people, though, are far more musical, more truly gifted, creative, and effective than they dare imagine.

What follows is a description of what we have found helpful at the A.C.C.: what we do and do not do. Much of it revolves, in various ways, around one remarkable man.

Vernon was a highly trained musician. As a young man he had studied for a career in classical music (while dreaming, secretly, of going on the stage). Although his great love was the organ, he also studied piano. As a young man, he had left college to take over the family business. He had played organ in churches over the years and had accompanied various school and community musicals on the piano.

As a result of his early training, Vernon retained an astonishing technique, including full chords on every note. He also had a remarkably extensive repertoire. He did not play by ear; if he didn't know it, then he couldn't play it. It may be significant that his ability to sight-read music, formerly impressive, had already become eroded (though his general reading ability was still quite good).

Vernon also had an electric sense of humor, an infectious love of performing (which to some extent blossomed in his dementia), a remarkable joie de vivre, vibrant energy, and curiosity. He loved to play for sing-alongs or to sit down with a band and lead the way. His performance pieces were minirecitals and tended not to be from the standard sing-along repertoire. Examples, performed with intensity and flair, included *Old Man River, How Deep Is the Ocean,* and *Stardust.* He played renditions of *I'll Be Seeing You* and *Somewhere over the Rainbow* that rarely left a dry eye in the vicinity. (Efforts by several volunteers to uncover, or resurrect, intact pieces of classical music revealed brilliant recalled flashes, but his "original," classical repertoire had apparently become extinguished.)

Vernon was a cornerstone of the facility's life. It is not exaggerating to say that he became something of a legend. Several factors did require more or less assistance: notably, his near-complete lack of short-term memory and extreme hearing deficit. He tended to play the same few songs repeatedly, to the point of annoying his peers. He also played extremely loudly. (With a hearing aid, his playing style changed dramatically and revealed further levels of his talent. Unfortunately, he loathed his hearing aid.)

Vernon always preferred up-tempo numbers. Because these, played with his power and volume, could be highly agitating in the late afternoon or evening, the staff needed to actively suggest appropriate numbers that he knew: *Moonlight Becomes You* as opposed to *Dark Town Strutters' Ball*. Certain songs, such as *Home on the Range*, became repeated, or perseverated, "loops" from which he needed assistance—and concerted effort—to exit.

Many of our most cherished A.C.C. memories involve Vernon. The songs we sing and love still reflect the wealth of music he shared with us, taught to us. If you know what to listen for, you can still hear his laugh in quiet corners. But eventually, Vernon's dementia began to make major inroads. He no longer independently thought of playing. Even his long-practiced musical skills eroded to the point that he experienced more frustration than enjoyment.

It was a major passage for the A.C.C. staff, volunteers, and family to confront the loss of this extraordinary friend. We were also more than a little apprehensive about the prospect of life without his music (even though he had been playing less often, for shorter periods, and with more malfunctions). As with any loss, we were not adequately prepared. And things certainly have not been the same. However, an interesting set of developments has taken place.

First, the number of musical volunteers has grown greatly. Some very willing musicians had simply assumed that we did not need them. Others admitted to having felt intimidated by Vernon's talent. Staff members suddenly realized how many lyrics we either had forgotten or had never bothered to learn. With Vernon, the words to songs mattered even less than usual, since they could rarely be heard. With him at the piano, we could all more less mumble along and it didn't make much difference.

Something began to become apparent: the power of a cappella singing. The beauty of voices blending together revealed itself. Many more folks sang to begin with; others sang more often and louder than they had before. Soft, simple, harmonies appeared in such old standards as *Love's Old Sweet Song, Beautiful Dreamer, In the Garden,* or *Abide with Me.*

Most group leaders (certainly this one) are painfully self-conscious about their own voices drifting around for anyone to hear. We all love the sound, however, when someone else leads the singing. And, regardless of how it might sound from outside the group, it feels wonderful—"like family"—from within.

Other challenges became apparent in Vernon's absence.

There is a common phenomenon with dementia: the tendency to accelerate. It might be compared to running downhill, gaining momentum. After a point, one either continues to go faster or loses balance altogether. This phenomenon is commonly observed during meals ("shoveling syndrome") and during walks, as noted in Chapter 5.

There is a musical and rhythmic equivalent. With dementia, the sense of rhythm often deteriorates; normal rhythms simply speed up. For want of a standardized term, I'll call it *dysrhythmia*. A strong instrument, such as the piano, or a strong leader with, say, a guitar, can keep folks in time pretty well. When singing unaccompanied, though, individuals start to have dysrhythmia sneak in. Unfortunately, singing a well-known song without its more or less normal beat, without the usual breaks or interludes, can be as difficult and annoying as singing known lyrics to an unknown tune.

A frequent example comes at the end of each verse of the *Battle Hymn of the Republic*. There is a seven-beat interlude before the chorus. Singers with dementia will tend to burst right through that pause. Such a lapse makes it difficult for others singing or humming to catch up or follow. And it gets faster; a song that started as a ballad will, if left unchecked, often end up sounding like "fast forward."

As with exercise programs, a group leader's voice is very important in maintaining control and direction (i.e., rhythm). Sometimes this means singing a little stronger or a little more loudly than a given (dysrhythmic) individual. It is also helpful for the leader to keep time by snapping fingers, clapping hands, or slapping the thigh. (But caution: clapping can sometimes overly increase the noise and energy levels.) Accentuating ("punching") terminal consonants in lyrics, especially at the end of each line, also aids in preserving a semblance of the song's natural rhythm (e.g., "Let me call you sweetheart," or "She'll be comin' round the mountain when she comes!")

A useful technique is for the group leader to begin each song very slowly, to hold or drag out the first word or two. By the second word, most folks will have chimed in. This establishes control and helps participants recognize the song. It also helps establish the key.

One early aspect of our program, utilizing Vernon's musical gifts and love of performing, was to conduct regular sing-along sessions at a neighborhood nursing home. Vernon was the star of the effort; between six and sixteen other folks would go along to visit and participate in the program. (This visiting group sometimes outnumbered the audience.)

The reactions of our visiting group after these sessions point out the importance of being needed; our residents and A.D.P. participants were functioning as volunteers and reaping the rewards. With Vernon, folks mingled a great deal with the nursing-home patients, sang along, danced, and socialized. They did not tend to congregate around the piano, and their singing was more or less incidental.

We had learned previously, on occasions when Vernon was ill, that a cappella sing-alongs away from home do not "translate." Fortunately, after Vernon left us, a talented volunteer agreed to take over the piano for the sing-outs. Despite her initial, understandable, worries about having a tough act to follow, these musical trips have continued to be of great value and benefit to our folks and to the residents of the nursing home.

Like the rest of our music, however, the sing-outs have changed. The focus is no longer on the piano and the pianist: it is on the singers. They suddenly became aware of being uncertain about lyrics—especially in public! My own function, accordingly, has changed. I formerly helped Vernon think of songs (and avoid playing *Over There* too many times: after all, many of the nursing-home residents do *not* have short-term memory deficits). Now I function more as a choir director. The group knows the song: I cue the words for them, as sort of a two-legged TelePrompTer. With that anchor of lyrical security, and with familiar tunes, they sing with gusto, cheer, and periodic harmony. They tend not to visit and cheer up the patients as much as they used to, however, at least not during the actual program.

Generally, singers with dementia cannot use lyric sheets. They tend to become bewildered, preoccupied with the competing cognitive tasks of reading and singing, and they tend to do neither. This dynamic would suggest caution in introducing someone with dementia to a karaoke machine.

• The Uses of Music •

The uses of music fall into four categories: program-oriented, entertainment, independent, and environmental.

Program-Oriented Music

Music has universal and near-constant value in structured dementia activity. The most obvious example is the frequent, often spontaneous singing that is a hallmark of most activity, be it with a large group (a group walk), with a small group (making sandwiches), one-to-one (making a bed), or independent ("happy wandering").

Most structured programs can incorporate music. Our use of music with exercise has been discussed. Songs can be used in any aspect of cognitive stimulation (sung, listened to, or both). Frequent uses include morning songs during a basic orientation ("morning almanac") session. Specific songs could help differentiate each day: if we're singing *Oh! How I Hate to Get Up in the Morning,* then it must be Monday.

Most theme discussions can incorporate musical tie-ins. Car songs would be indispensable to "old auto" discussions; school songs, to "school days." No focus group on moose would be complete without a few traditional "moose" songs (Moose *over Miami, When the* Moose *Comes over the Mountain,* etc.). Numerous birth-date salutes suggest themselves, such as Kate Smith, Bing Crosby, Judy Garland—even, to a lesser degree, Elvis. Musical tie-ins with specific places—California, the Mississippi, Scotland, the South—are staples of activity programs. Connections with holiday discussions are as common as they are productive.

The "simple" process of singing or humming along may well be the most valuable cognitive therapy of all, besides laughing.

Entertainment

Entertainment usually implies live music—music that is not related to a specific program but *is* a program in and of itself. It implies volunteers, who may well be residents themselves. Musical entertainment has been a cornerstone of activity programing in long-term care for as long as there have been long-term care facilities. (Alexander the Great insisted on musicians and singers for his hospitals, along with homelike "therapeutic" gardens.)

One immediate difference in programing musical and other entertainment for the dementia setting is that programs must fit the needs of the residents and, within reason, their natural daily pattern. For example, many wonderful musical programs are conducted in various facilities during the evening. Evening programs are not merely convenient for those donating their time and talents but also necessary, in order to assemble the more or less large numbers of volunteers involved. Such musical programs tend to be inappropriate for the dementia setting. To begin with, individuals are often more prone, after dark or after a day of being busy, to perceptions of being "invaded" ("Who are all these people? I didn't invite them into my house. Get them out!") More important, while large, high-energy programs may be greatly enjoyed while in progress, the level of energy tends to stay high long after the entertainers go home—all night long, in some cases.

This is not to say that all evening programs should be avoided. "Quiet" entertainments, brief (20–30 minutes) and presented by small groups, can be appreciated and well tolerated.

Similar precautions pertain to late afternoon as well. And any large or loud program, even in the morning, should have special measures taken afterward. There should never be a sudden vacuum, of either music or energy, just as one should never exercise vigorously and then suddenly stop without some cool-down period. Change should never be sudden. Serving a snack is often helpful, as well as being quite socially normal. Quiet but similar music on the stereo may help everyone to shift gears.

Some very high quality entertainment tends to be uncommonly disturbing. As mentioned in Chapter 5, certain sopranos, especially singing solo, can sound "screechy" to the person with dementia, while in fact singing well and beautifully. Violinists can have the same effect (though fiddlers rarely do). Some instruments, notably the piano (especially played honky-tonk style), tend to be agitatingly loud.

Sheer volume is less important than the quality, the timbre, of the music. A brass quintet (trombones and tuba) proved to be surprisingly effective, even relaxing (and even in the evening).

Other programs, musical or not, can present the opposite dilemma. Puppet shows, while visually engaging, often have muffled dialogue and sound effects. Young kids' plays and skits are notoriously hard to hear; pure cuteness goes only so far with abridged attention spans.

Amplifiers should be avoided, if only to avoid the inevitable—and inevitably "catastrophizing"—problems with shrieking feedback. Many excellent musicians feel unnecessarily wedded to their mike and amp. Most electrified instruments, such as guitars, are generally inappropriate to begin with. (Let's hope we never have to know how music by Jimi Hendrix or Keith Richards or Eric Clapton mixes with dementia, when it comes to be age-appropriate.)

Independent/Individual Music

The most obvious independent use of music is simply listening. If folks with dementia could tolerate wearing a Walkman with earplugs, then independent use of music would increase dramatically.

The vehicle for most individual enjoyment of music is naturally the portable radio or tape player. Some folks, for example, benefit from selected music at their bedside, whether they are ill, taking a nap, or enjoying quiet time in their room. Some individuals benefit from "sleepy" music, such as lullabies, at bedtime; others start searching for their mother or their own babies.

A fairly frequent request (from folks who can still make them) is for more classical music. We often forget, today, that classical music, recordings, and performances were as much a part of everyday life fifty and seventy-five years ago as "top 40" radio or MTV is today.

One gentleman was a native of Vienna, Austria. His transition to the A.C.C. was difficult. A thoughtful aide discovered that a tape of Strauss waltzes created for him a sense of being at home in his new room.

Environmental Music

When music is not used in any of the above ways, then it is usually used as a component of the environment. This often means using music as a mood-affecting tool.

Music, above all, should never overload the aural environment like television that nobody is watching. Music should never add to the "static," the auditory clutter already in the air.

A dementia environment, by definition, is a quiet place. Mixed sounds create chaos, and chaos is always agitating. (Picture the typical child-rearing household at five o'clock in the afternoon.) Music should never create chaos and should never make chaos worse. If music is clashing with sound from a television, then chaos prevails, even if in a limited area. In this case, either a door should be shut or one or the other of the sources of sound should be eliminated (or at least turned down). If there is music playing and a vacuum cleaner suddenly roars to life, then either the music should be turned off or the vacuuming should be postponed.

Music should also match the prevailing mood. If the goal after a dance is to lower the general energy level, to induce quiet, then the perfect number to play first on a tape would be another dance number, preferably in a style not unlike the departing band. It could be a waltz as opposed to a tango, but should not be the Lucarelli's magic oboe playing *Pavane for a Dead Princess*. (A bit of "environmental dissonance" before a band starts playing may be more or less unavoidable. Even folks watching the musicians set up and tune their instruments may be jolted when the music actually starts. As always, the staff needs to be alert to individuals likely to have traumatic reactions. On the other hand, playing background music to prepare folks may backfire: background music plus real instruments is certain chaos.)

Music is a valuable tool but rarely works on its own. That is, if the goal is to induce a "sleepy" mood, a Quiet Hour, then the staff needs to work along with the music to assist folks in quieting down. One can't just "slap on a tape," however appropriate it might be, walk away, and expect a somnolent mood to happen automatically. "Quiet" does not imply the absence of staff. But once tranquillity is achieved, music can certainly help suggest that everyone remain that way.

What music, then, is relaxing to the ear with dementia? In the first place, music follows the basic rules: the most relaxing music will be familiar to the individual. The more familiar, the more homey it will feel. Beyond that, the mood of the music should be quiet: *There's a Long, Long Trail*, as opposed to *Put on Your Old Gray Bonnet*.

The tempo should be slow. In musical terms, the mood should be largo, as opposed to allegro. The Andante movement from *The William Tell Overture* makes ideal relaxation music. If only because of its traditional use as morning music, it's especially good before breakfast: awakening, relaxing, and orienting as well. It is, however, followed by the frenetic *Lone Ranger Theme*, which, bursting in as it does, would be sufficient to drive most any breakfast crowd to distraction.

The fewer notes, the better. Chord structures should be unornamented. Most music from the Baroque period tends to be uniquely disturbing to the ear with dementia. One gentleman, a retired Fortune 500 executive, had historically preferred two pieces by Mozart for relaxation: Piano Concerto no. 26 and Concerto for Flute and Harp in C Major. But played as background in our library while he peacefully read, the pieces agitated him. A Quiet Hour tape proved effective.

The timbre should be low, unlike that of the "screechy" violin and unlike that of the highly touted flute, which all too often fails to soothe.

The instrumentation should be in a low register. Low violin can be calming; low cello can be more so.

The fewer instruments and the simpler the sound, the more reliably relaxing the music.

The changes between notes within the tune should be gradual. Sudden jumps should be avoided. Even the Brahms lullaby contains a full-octave leap that, on violin or flute, can be disconcerting.

It should be added that the tune, even if familiar and all-of-the-above, should not be innately disturbing. Neither *Home Sweet Home* nor the traditional funeral dirge, the Chopin "Funeral March Sonata" (Sonata no. 2 in B-flat Minor, op. 35, third movement, *Marche Funebre*), would be a wise bet to induce relaxation.

The perfect dementia relaxation music, then, would be a slow, familiar, nonprovocative melody, with one-step intervals, set in a low register, and played by an oboe or a bassoon. Candidates include the inevitable Pachelbel Canon, the Albinoni Adagio, and the Largo from Dvorak's *New World* Symphony.

Most of the recorded music that we use at the A.C.C. has been specially made (home taped). The tapes are mostly programed, or dedicated, compilations of one sort or another. CDs (at least at this writing) do not give us the same flexibility, so they are seldom used. Record players, too, pose many problems, some of which spawned the CD fad to begin with: brief play-time, scratches, skips, the required storage space, the low probability that the records would be returned to their jackets, and so on. Tape players are also cheaper.

Generally, we do not use background music if an activity is in progress. This includes meals, during which music tends to have a disruptive effect. Relaxing music during work sessions (table activities) may not be disturbing, but any background noise during discussions can be deadly. Nevertheless, there are times when music helps weave a social atmosphere, especially at functions like late-afternoon teas and ice cream socials. No Happy Hour can long exist without something in the background (if only Boots Randolph). Live music during any of these can be a wonderful addition: a solo flute or cello or harmonica, for instance. One way or another, we often sing our way into supper (and lunch too, for that matter), leaving a more or less brief quiet period before the actual meal.

• A Few Unrelaxing Musical Things to Avoid •

- Synthesized music.
  It tends to be less relaxing than acoustic music.
- Any single type of recorded music for more than a half-hour.
  A solid hour of music might pass, but only if varied. Too much
  of anything is too much, be it Patsy Cline, Bing Crosby, or the
  Mormon Tabernacle Choir.
- Nature tapes.
  Wind means there's a storm; seagulls sound like wailing babies;
  crashing surf feels disorienting if you're inland; babbling
  brooks (at best) sound like burst plumbing; a swarm of cica-
  das in the living room is a disturbing development; jungle
  sounds might as well come from Mars.
- Rhythm bands.
  Most of the sounds produced are precisely perfect to drive an
  ear with dementia to distraction, especially those not directly
  involved but within earshot. In live performances they often
  come across as infantile and rarely sound musical in any way.
- "Top 40" radio, of any variety.
  Most pop music is targeted to an audience barely beyond pu-
  berty. The way to stay young at heart is not to have one's
  senses assaulted by alien music.
- Any other radio.
  Once turned on, a radio, like a television, tends to stay on. Inter-
  ruptions for news, announcements, and much louder advertising are as disruptive and disturbing as an intercom system.
  Too often, this is a lazy and inefficient way of controlling the
  environment.
- Anyone "plunking" a piano—especially energetic children.

• The Therapeutic Pedestal •

I had often wished for a rolling stool for sing-alongs. It always seemed
that such a thing would make eye contact, and getting to eye level,
much easier. It would make it easier to lead people, to work with individuals and with the whole group, without constant standing, stoop-
ing, bending, and even "duck walking." (The leader's standing up from

a chair can give an unintended visual cue to the group to do likewise.) I had tried various rolling chairs, with and without armrests, but a stool seemed like the ideal thing. Unfortunately, suitable models were prohibitively expensive.

It happened that our secretary obtained a much-needed new desk chair. The back rest of her old chair was falling apart. I took it, as my own desk chair was quite low and would be well suited for residents to sit in while in my office. The back rest, however, grew increasingly wobbly and began to drop nuts and bolts.

One day, Tony was exceptionally anxious to "find his brothers and get back to work." He was outside my office and on the verge of getting into an altercation with another resident. A former carpenter and all-around handy person, Tony was usually willing to help out. "O.K., O.K.," he grumbled to my request for assistance. "But just quick, I'm a hurry!"

I showed him my chair, pointed out where the nuts and bolts had fallen out, and shrugged. He proceeded to turn the chair upside down, gestured for tools (which were nearby in a desk drawer), and began to take the back rest apart.

It took about twenty minutes. Tony decided that I needed some parts; I said I'd get them. He then insisted that, since he had helped me, I should help him find his brothers and get back to work!

The next time I needed something to engage Tony, I arrayed the chair and its parts and asked him for help once again. Again, he agreed to help. However, we could not reassemble the chair precisely as it had been.

Eventually we would have needed a welding torch to repair that chair's back rest. However, a new therapeutic tool had revealed itself: a rolling, swiveling stool. And it has been as valuable as I'd thought.

• A Bad Idea •

There's nothing like the sound of running water to trigger urinary urgency. One day, in the interest of making the resident assistant's task at toileting time a bit easier, and not heeding one wise co-worker's misgivings, I played a tape which featured a "relaxing" babbling brook. It worked wonders. Never before (or, luckily, since) had there been such a rush to the toilets. The staff bathroom was pressed into service. The tide of extreme urgency could not be stemmed. Chaos ensued.

One gentleman was quite agitated. Not, as it turned out, because he had to urinate, but because he couldn't find the burst water pipes he thought he was hearing. His frustration was sharpened because the bathrooms were all full of women!

• Our Favorite Songs •

A Baker's Dozen of Popular Standards

1. *Let Me Call You Sweetheart*
2. *It's a Long, Long, Way to Tipperary*
3. *Down by the Old Mill Stream*
4. *You Are My Sunshine*
5. *My Wild Irish Rose, When Irish Eyes Are Smiling*
6. *Over There*
7. *Darktown Strutter's Ball*
8. *Daisy Bell (Daisy, Daisy)*
   This song lends itself especially well to role-playing; it originally had wonderfully sentimental verses.
9. *Jingle Bells*
   Originally a winter song, it has nothing, technically, to do with
   Christmas. It can be effective (and fun) in a July heat wave.
   The several verses suggest possibilities for both discussion
   and role-playing or dramatization.
10. *Shine on, Harvest Moon*
    Common courtesy demands that we discuss the old-fashioned
    terms "croon" and "spoon."
11. *The Man on the Flying Trapeze*
    A good example of old, storytelling (and high dramatic) verses.
12. *Yes! We Have No Bananas*
    A huge sing-along favorite in its day (c. 1923), it combines a
    very familiar verse with nearly endless, absurdly funny
    verses.

A Baker's Dozen of Our Favorite Folk Songs

Folk songs are particularly valuable: they are ancient; they are repetitive; they are very rhythmic; they have very singable melodies; they

were learned in childhood. They can also lend themselves to endless improvisation. And they can be very humorous.

The most familiar part of most songs is naturally the chorus. Familiarity—and participation—can be maximized by singing the chorus after every verse.

1. *I've Been Working on the Railroad*

2. *Clementine*

   Suggests various pantomime possibilities. For example, Clem's size-nine feet, her clumsiness (the "splinter" was clearly a small tree trunk), and the last verse, in which the heartbroken boyfriend admits, "Then I kissed her older [less ageist than *little*] sister, and forgot my Clementine!" There is a potentially morbid side to this song. I like to add that Clem actually swam across "the water" and ran off to California, where she lived happily ever after; the verse about her fertilizing "rosies and other posies" can also be edited to good effect.

3. *He's Got the Whole World in His Hands*

   This is one of the newer numbers in our traditional repertoire. What He has in His hands—and who—can vary endlessly, including individual names, the weather, food items, pets, famous people, participants' names, and so on.

4. *Skip to My Lou*

   This magically familiar tune not only tells the sad story of the young man whose date jilted him at the big dance but also lends itself to a rhyming closure game: words that rhyme with "Lou." As written, the lyrics usually are "Little Red Wagon, painted blue," "Flies in the buttermilk, shoofly shoe," etc. Additions could include "On our feet we wear two shoes," "If you get a cold, you'll go 'A-choo!'" "Planted a seed; it grew and grew," and so on, more or less indefinitely.

5. *Jimmy Crack Corn (The Blue Tail Fly)*

6. *Oh, Susannah!*

   One of the unique qualities of this song is the nonsense (non sequitur, hyperbolic) lyrics. A typical adaptation, to add even more repetition, is to break and sing the chorus half-way through the verse (after "Susannah for to see"). Musically, the coda is simply ignored in each verse. The result is twice as many "Oh, Susannah"s!

7. *When the Saints Go Marching In*

   There is definitely a spiritual, uplifting quality to this song. Alternative lyrics could include almost any idea: "And when the sun/decides to shine (Then we all want to be in that number)," "When we all/are feeling great," "When our lunch/is finally cooked," etc.

8. *The Green Grass Grew All Around*

   By whatever name, this can be the ultimate ad-lib song. It can emphasize closure and short-term recall in a very nonthreatening way. The noun at the end of each verse is simply dropped: "And on that tree/there was a . . . (What?)" Before long, somebody will offer a "thing," and it gets added to the incremental list. The list is never the same twice.

9. *She'll Be Comin' Round the Mountain*

   This can be used as a communal story, deciding on what steps to take to greet her, "when she comes." The standard nursing home sing-along version, with additions and motions ("Whoa, back," with motions of pulling on reins; "Chop! Chop!" to "kill the old red rooster," etc.), which then adds each addition to those preceding, has special uses with a memory-impaired group.

10. *The Old Gray Mare*

    It somehow seems less than encouraging to hear a group of elderly people singing, "She ain't what she used to be/many long years ago." It is interesting to watch folks' reactions if the words are changed to "She's better than she used to be!" Verses can be added, explaining how the old horse is an improvement on her younger self (for example, she could be quieter, smarter, wiser, calmer, etc.).

11. *Froggie Went a-Courtin'*

    This song exists in many variations. Most include one, nearly mystical feature: the "Uh-huh" repeated in the chorus. This has become a touchstone at the A.C.C. Folks repeat it independently and surprisingly. One nonverbal lady learned and repeatedly used the "Uh-huh" to great comical effect. It seems possible that the abdominal nature of the "Uh-huh" expostulation creates a unique effect. (The designers of an advertising blitz for a certain popular cola clearly thought so.)

12. *The Red River Valley*

13. *Billy Boy*

A Baker's Dozen of Our Favorite Hymns

1. *I Love to Tell the Story*
2. *The Old Rugged Cross*
3. *Blessed Assurance*
4. *God Be with You Till We Meet Again.*
5. *In the Garden*
6. *What a Friend We Have in Jesus*
7. *Amazing Grace*
8. *How Great Thou Art*
9. *When the Roll Is Called up Yonder*
10. *May the Good Lord Bless and Keep You*
11. *The Church in the Wildwood*
12. *It Is No Secret*
13. *Just a Closer Walk with Thee*

A Baker's Dozen of Patriotic Songs

We recall that there was a time when children learned our "national" songs in school, and typically began each day with at least one selection. Examples naturally begin with:

1. *The Star-Spangled Banner*
2. *Yankee Doodle*
3. *America the Beautiful*
4. *America (My Country 'tis of Thee)*
5. *Columbia! The Gem of the Ocean!*
6. *God Bless America* (We do need to be aware that this number, unlike the difficult-to-sing *Star-Spangled Banner*, invariably triggers a reaction of standing up.
7. *The Battle Hymn of the Republic* (This melody, like that of our national anthem, was a drinking song long before Julia Ward Howe wrote her memorable lyrics, even before John Brown

grew a beard. Kids still sing, and create, alternative sets of words to the tune.)

8. *Dixie*
9. *You're a Grand Old Flag*
10. *The Battle Cry of Freedom*
11. *When Johnny Comes Marching Home*
12. *Over There!*
13. *Praise the Lord and Pass the Ammunition!*

A Baker's Dozen of Good Relaxing Tapes and Records

1. *A Journey Home,* Kelly/Bogdanovic (Harp & Guitar), Global Pacific Records GPC 337
2. *O'Carolan's Dream,* Patrick Ball (Celtic Harp), Fortuna Records 17061-4
3. *Nocturne* (*Music for a Romantic Evening*), Anthology, Cameo Classics, The Moss Music Group CC 1025 (One of those cassettes typically found in bookstores.)
4. *Stress Busters* (*Music for a Stressless World*), RCA Victor 09026-60710-4
5. *The Pachelbel Canon and other Baroque Favorites,* Allegro, Moss Music Group ACS 8098. The first side of this is ideal; the second side, Bach's Brandenburg Concerto No. 5, is not.
6. *Good Morning,* Steven Halpern, SRX. I spied this tape in a dark corner of a music store and bought it on a whim. The "free-floating" piano music seemed a definite improvement over an earlier, synthesized relaxation effort. After a few weeks of consistent and effective use, one fact became clear: it certainly had a calming, morale-raising effect on the staff!
7. *The Relaxing Magic of the Oboe,* Lucarelli, Heartland Music HC1046. Anthologies of oboe music contain a variety of pieces, usually not geared specifically toward relaxation.
8. *A Return to Romance,* Zamfir, PolyGram 836 056-4
9. *It's So Peaceful in the Country,* Percy Faith Orchestra with Mitch Miller on Oboe (Instrumental), Columbia CL 779
10. *Nightfall,* Carmen Dragon (Instrumental collection), Capitol Records P 8575

11. *Dreamland (The Sleep Tape)*, Scott Fitzgerald Nature Recordings, Vol. XIX

12. *A Rainbow Path*, Kay Gardiner, Ladyslipper, Inc. LRC 103. This and related recordings are fascinating explorations of the uses of music in healing and health. While some selections may sound a bit "alien" to the ear with dementia, most have a notable calming effect on residents and staff alike.

13. *Goodnight, Amadeus*, Silo Records MLP 2108. Programed classical music to relax kids—or the rest of us—to sleep.

Note: Various recording companies have at one time or another produced collections of music to relax by, ranging from single albums to monumental collections (such as by *Reader's Digest*). This effort seems to have been particularly common during the late 1950s. It is difficult to spend much time around used records without coming across more examples than you would care to. Many are, in fact, worth investing the 50 cents at the yard sale, if only to tape from: Nothing ventured, nothing gained!

·: 7 :·

Art

Much of the literature regarding the value of art as a therapy and as an activity for people with dementia treat it as another aspect of therapeutic arts, healing arts, cultural arts, and so on. This is certainly a dementia-appropriate approach. However, many aspects set the visual arts apart.

First, and perhaps foremost, is the fact that art—drawing, painting, and so on—is relatively alien to many individuals. For folks born, say, before 1930, art is not generally a part of everyday life. Exercise, work, humor, music, language use, even aspects of play may be integral aspects of people's lives; art, though, to a large extent is not. This is especially true in terms of active participation: actually painting, drawing, etc. Few automatic skills, either verbal or physical, will be triggered by art exercises.

Interest in art centers on the possibilities it offers for self-expression. Dementia will almost inevitably rob the individual of self-expression through the usual channels: speaking, writing, singing, etc. The possibility that visual arts may help re-open expressive channels or help slow the process of being cut off is very appealing.

Literature on dementia and art often focuses on specific individuals. Some life-long and/or professional artists have retained their sense of self through adaptations: therapeutic interventions, often on a one-to-one basis with helpers, have assisted them to retain but alter their art as the dementia progresses. Others have "discovered" joy and self-expression through one expressive channel or another, not uncommonly in situations where a great deal of one-to-one support is available. The writing, rather notably, tends to focus at least as much on the therapist as on the person with dementia: the artist's progress of learning, of coping with, say, Alzheimer disease; the joy of helping individuals unlock their inner doors. Unhappily, few programs can afford to pay a professional art therapist, even on a part-time basis.

Be that as it may, there is a unique value to art; it has unique effects on participants. Sudden and surprising miracles abound. The impact of, say, painting, may well surpass our ability to gauge or comprehend it: it is ultimately personal, and largely nonverbal.

It may be that specific knowledge of materials, techniques, and therapeutic principles is more important with art than with other therapies. This does not mean, however, that the effective use of art is beyond the ability of "unartistic" caregivers, whether at home or in a group setting.

Over the years, at the A.C.C., we have dabbled with many art-oriented techniques. Most of the staff and residents have or have raised children and were naturally intrigued by the possibilities of adapting activities that they had effectively used at home to the individuals they were working with. These ranged from cartooning (as a "watching" activity), to illustrating group-created stories, to using prints of familiar paintings as discussion topics. Techniques ranged from "instant painting" coloring books (in which the colors emerge as you brush on water); to free-form drawing groups using markers, crayons, and water-color trays; to finger painting; to by-the-number "black velvet" kits. No such efforts were without interest, and there were some fascinating results. None, however, seemed to have an impact on more than a handful of individuals; none seemed to light a blaze of enthusiasm, of promise. Some, such as repeated efforts with fingerpaints, were notably ineffective.

After a time, we obtained a small grant to purchase art supplies and to offer a small stipend to a consultant. The goal was to determine which projects and materials could be easily utilized by the staff, both during organized sessions and on an as-needed basis. We wanted to find out what worked, how to conduct specific activities, and whom they benefited. The search was, in part, for the "lowest common denominators" in terms of group involvement and impact on individuals.

The results of early sessions were mixed. Each session consisted of several different projects, to allow maximal flexibility of cognitive level and individual interest. We kept track of which projects were promising and which participants were particularly engaged.

Then, the paints came. When folks first touched brush to paint, then to paper, a magic started to flow. The results were dramatic. Some tried to represent an object on the table; some simply watched the brush, calling on some unseen source, almost like consulting a Ouija board.

The process of painting continues to be extraordinarily engaging. Smiles often occur immediately; moods turn more cheerful. Spontaneous singing often occurs. Two otherwise difficult-to-involve men have remained engaged, with rapt attention, for an hour and more. Individuals begin reminiscing: "My sister could draw awful good"; "My father painted, and he taught me—a long time ago!" These memories tend to be the same each session.

Clarice has been quite involved in most art sessions. She will never sit down and draw or paint if asked, but once she begins doing so on her own, she will often work with wonderful task-attentiveness. Her long-term memory is quite clear, and she can express it very well. Her short-term recall, however, even minute-to-minute, is virtually nonexistent. Clarice mentioned that her brother used to draw. With some coaching or prompting, she explained, "He could draw anything—so real, lifelike. But it got him in trouble. Once, he drew my mother: it looked just like her. But didn't she get cross! She was a heavy woman, and he drew all her chins!"

Ira was a day-care participant. After a few initial visits, he was usually fairly calm, happy to participate in any group program. His primary focus was on the time, and specifically the time when his wife was due to pick him up. He generally declined to "help out" with any work- or task-type activity.

Asked to join a sketching group one day, he scoffed, "I can't do any of that," and laughed. He did sit with the group, though, and observed. After about twenty minutes, he picked up a colored marker and started sketching. He worked very attentively for another half hour, eventually used three colors, and produced quite an interesting treatment of the vase of flowers on the table.

Ira's recollections of day care were rarely accurate, though usually positive. In relating what he did during the day, he would typically confabulate beautifully but usually without much relation to what had actually gone on. One evening, several days after this art session, a family member overheard Ira talking to his granddaughter on the phone. Apparently answering a question about day care, he said, "Oh yeah, I go there days, to the club. To help out. And you won't believe: they've got me drawing! And not bad, either!"

• Bernie's Story •

One resident, Bernie, had been a professional artist. His work is in several well-known museums; he had taught at an Ivy League college. He had written several widely read books, and at least one book has been written (by another author) about his own work.

Bernie and his wife, Kay, had long summered in Maine and had always planned to retire to their cottage. He had retired two years earlier; in fact, earlier than planned. He had already started to show signs of an obvious dementia: having always had a good memory for students' names, he now was not only forgetting them but identifying them as students from his first few years of teaching. He kept writing and rewriting the same scholarly article, with no recollection that he had even started work on it before. He threw out an entire class's papers.

Bernie had done little painting during the past few years, but in the decade or so before that, his style had grown less representational, more abstract. His renowned technique grew less precise. His wife commented that she hated to look at the later work. "It terrifies me," she confided. Bernie had undergone extensive diagnostic testing, which had included an MRI. When Kay saw the results of the test, she wept. "The test results looked like those paintings," she explained. "He hadn't been painting in an abstract style; he had been painting pictures of his dementia. It's as if he'd been painting a scan of his brain."

The family had cautioned us not to expect Bernie to participate in groups, and he didn't. Moreover, he thought most group activities were demeaning, an insult to his intelligence.

One day Bernie surprised me by listening, at a distance, to a discussion for a few minutes. I tried to gear the discussion a bit more toward him: rather than choosing words with as few syllables as possible, I inserted a few more sophisticated terms. He seemed very attentive, and appeared intrigued. Then he actually spoke. I was thrilled. His sentence faltered half-way through; I knew better than to attempt to cue, or re-feed, his words to him. After a moment, I simply acknowledged what he had said, attempted to paraphrase it, and thanked him.

"Yes," he replied in a scathing tone, standing up. "'Thanks'—for not much!" He strode off in a dramatic whirl, and told a volunteer, "This is utter nonsense . . . like the third grade."

Even before Bernie's admission, I had been searching for a special volunteer: an artist, or at least someone with a love and knowledge of art. That search, aided by an area volunteer agency, was successful: the volunteer was a retired physician who was enjoying a new career with watercolor landscapes and was more or less familiar with Bernie's work. His efforts to get Bernie to paint or draw, though, were not successful. The volunteer led several demonstration groups, which Bernie joined as an "expert consultant" (although he was resentful of any time the volunteer spent with other residents or with staff members).

We tried to interest Bernie in helping out with group art projects, both with and without the volunteer. Even when not jealous of his friend, though, Bernie deemed the groups "infantile" and the participants "idiots." He did enjoy watching the volunteer sketch, around our grounds and outside of the facility and on one occasion in his home studio. They enjoyed visits to local galleries, usually followed by lunch together. Bernie would recall having gone to a "show," though he would not realize if they visited the same gallery over again. These lunches out stopped when eating in public became too frustrating for Bernie, but he was equally glad to have the volunteer join him, at a private table, for lunch at our facility.

Bernie's dementia continued to progress rapidly. Toward the end of his time at the A.C.C., he would become extremely upset in almost any group setting. One of the few activities that occupied him was sitting in my office (the "library") and perusing the book about his artwork. He would look through the prints of his paintings and make comments like, "That's nice," or "Good color," or "Interesting." He had no idea that the paintings were his own.

• Some General Principles •

Some general principles for art activities have become apparent.

Above all, whatever the project or whatever tools are being used, the emphasis must be on the process, not the finished product. One lady spent a good forty-five minutes one day, painting what she referred to as people. She then, rather suddenly, began to cover the entire paper with broad strokes of color. She worked on that for another twenty minutes, until the whole thing was a mass of blue. She was very pleased with the result, and left with a feeling of optimism that lingered through the rest of the afternoon. Art had been truly therapeutic for her: she had been calm, happy, and involved and had even had carry-over emotion.

It is essential for the group leaders to be flexible, to "go with the flow," and to have a "palette" of ideas to fall back on.

The most motivating lines have been, "We're trying out some paints. Please come help us," or "We're trying an experiment. Will you help, please?"

One-to-one support is usually needed to help each participant get going, to find an appropriate task and to get into a "groove." It's best to start small, then build up—the Tom Sawyer method of motivation. If a small group starts to work and appears to be having a good time, and if the work itself has an interesting quality, then others will come naturally. Start with one or two tables, then add others one by one. If there are enough staff members helping, each could take a table or two. As the session progresses, the individuals at a given table might end up working on different projects, even in different media: one painting freehand, one painting an outlined picture, one stamping, and one rolling clay.

Precisely what each participant will do on a given day is not predictable. What is generally predictable, though, is the engagement.

Folks with dementia tend not to like things that are messy (as in cooking). Fingerpainting and string art have been nearly disastrous, not only because people were less than intrigued but also because, disturbed by the mess, they got up and left in a hurry. With painting, the inevitable paint on hands washes off easily—sometimes several times per session. Often, folks are so intent on what they're doing, though, that they don't notice until they're finished.

Items should be brightly colored (e.g., tempera as opposed to water-color paints).

Items should be easy to manipulate. Homemade clay dough is better than commercial clay, which is often very stiff and hard to soften up. Potters' clay, being quite messy, might be too far the other way.

Everything should be nontoxic. There is always at least one individual who will attempt to drink the paint water, use a paintbrush as lipstick, or devour the clay. Simple snack items should be on hand for individuals attempting to eat nonfood items. If fruit is being used to draw from, then it could be used as such a substitute.

Items should not be infantile. A coloring picture of a duck should be of a duck, not a "duckie"; a deer should be a deer, not Bambi.

All activities should be easy for the staff to prepare, conduct, and clean up after.

Projects and materials should be comfortable for the staff to use. Even those who might claim that they "can't draw a straight line" should be able to feel competent.

All items should be relatively inexpensive and easy to replace.

• A Baker's Dozen of Basic Art Supplies to Have on Hand •

An art program could be started simply, effectively, and inexpensively with just the first four of these items.

1. Good tempera paints, mostly in basic colors. We have found that cakes or trays work best (the trays for individuals who wish to use more than one color).
2. A variety of brushes (medium and fine, of fair to good quality).
3. Decent art paper (not necessarily expensive, but heavy enough not to buckle).
4. Large pads of newsprint, for drawing on and to cover tables. (Newspapers can be very distracting. Cut-open lawn-sized garbage bags are useful, and of course waterproof, although they may frighten some individuals: they make the table "disappear" or become a "hole.") Another way to protect tables is to use brightly colored vinyl tablecloths or table covers.
5. Construction paper.
6. Clay or homemade play-dough, kept on hand and ready to go.
7. Simple cookie cutters, seashells, and other basic geometric shapes (of wood, plastic, etc.).
8. Any good crayons.
9. Colored marker pens.
10. Ink pads (nonindelible) and assorted stamps.
11. (Safe) Scissors.

12. (Art) Tissue paper
13. Plaster Gauze ("O.C.L." strips)

• A Baker's Dozen of Art Ideas (Things to Try) •

1. Painting "free form."

   The simplest painting of all: simply give people a brush, paper, and water, with an object (or objects) on the table. "Help us see if this paint is any good," or ". . . what the colors look like", may be a more motivating "line" than "Come paint these flowers." Some individuals might do better with a half sheet, or even a quarter sheet, of paper. Some may be intimidated by a blank sheet of paper, though, and might be offered coloring sheets.

2. Coloring sheets.

   Simple outlines of plants, flowers, houses, antique cars, farm animals, etc. A good source of these, in reproducible form, is the Dover Catalogue (see Appendix B).

3. Stamps/stamp pads.

   Some individuals enjoy the repetitive activity of stamping. It does take two steps, but it is immediately gratifying. (This is similar to the common busywork activity of stamping envelopes—for real or not.)

4. Simple pottery, with clay or home-made flour dough.

   Pinch pots or coil pots are engaging for some. Once dried, they can be painted or otherwise decorated. (This is typically done in winter holiday time, with seasonal cookie cutters.)

5. Shape tracing.

   Tracing around basic geometric shapes is a fairly automatic function. Items should be roughly hand-sized. Shapes without corners (circles, ovals, hearts, fish, etc.) work best. A common project with children is tracing hands. Tracing one's own hand can be difficult for participants with dementia, but some would enjoy having a "helper" trace their hands, then painting or decorating them themselves. Hands copied by photocopier tend not to look like hands, and even can be frightening. Part of the problem may be the dark background produced around the copied hand. These shapes can then be used by the same worker, saved for another session, or passed on to another group member for painting shapes.

6. Painting shapes.

Individuals sometimes do well if given one or more simple shapes on a sheet of paper (drawn, traced, or photocopied). Or each participant may choose a shape or two. What each individual does with the shape(s) will depend on what he or she perceives at that moment. An egg, for example, may become a face; two eggs might become eyes; lines might become tree trunks. Or, very likely, observers may not know quite what they're seeing.

7. Partial faces.

Some will enjoy "finishing" a face if given, for example, the hair and two eyes, or two eyes and a nose.

8. Mixing colors ("color wheel").

A standard exercise for students of all ages: simply mixing basic colors and producing secondary colors (perhaps just two or three per session). The process may be very engaging; the colors may suggest interesting patterns and ideas.

9. "Crazy shapes."

Participants take a pencil, marker, or other device and, with eyes closed (and probably a little help from a friend), let one hand draw random lines, a design, on paper. They then decorate or paint it according to their fancy.

10. Torn paper collage.

This old standby can be effective, especially with two adaptations. First, the paper should be cut, or torn, as a separate project. Second, glue is messy, especially if using it on small, torn pieces of construction or tissue paper. Self-stick paper, or even contact paper, is easier and less messy to use. ("Crunch" art has proven a bit beyond our folks' capabilities: the added step of crunching, or rolling up, the paper presents the problem.)

11. Signature

Have each participant sign his or her work. This is often a very separate project. Sometimes the signature is much larger than the art itself. Some individuals will experience frustration in attempting a signature, whether with a brush or a pencil. Some, though, will be able to sign their names with a

paintbrush who cannot do so with a pen. One gentleman—
Milton—had lost most of his ability to speak. He understood
the task but had difficulty initiating his signature. He clearly
said "No" to hand-over-hand help. With perseverance,
though, and a lot of oral encouragement, Milton finally began to write—and did a passable job: writing, quite legibly,
"John Hancock."

12. "Plaster" Art.

Any object covered with strips of plaster gauze (O.C.L.) forms a
very spontaneous "sculpture." Balloons are a common example: the balloon is popped once the plaster has dried and
the shape is left to be painted or otherwise decorated.

13. Sketching/Doodling.

Simply given blank sheets of paper, individuals may sketch a given
object. Others, rather naturally, may simply start doodling.

·: 8 :·

Television and Videotapes

Television is not the complete evil that it has sometimes been assumed to be for people with dementia. As noted in Chapter 1, it can be a useful tool and a valuable activity resource. As the half-kidding joke goes, as a tranquilizer, TV is certainly more humane than most drugs.

Most network television presents the same problems as radio, with the obvious addition of visual considerations. In general, and with "dementia common sense," most quiz programs should be avoided: they are nightmares of noise. The topics of many talk shows are often bewildering, if not disturbing. The same often applies to the verbal violence on soap operas. Most situation comedies aren't funny, despite the laugh track; most dramas are either dull, violent, or both. Most children's shows look childish.

The best televiewing for people with dementia (and maybe for most of the rest of us, as well) tends to be reruns: "Golden Oldies," whether individual programs, such as in the early evening, or entire network programing, such as on an all-movie channel. In thinking about using television and videos, remember the principle of the "captive audience": the fact that folks will watch a given show is not an indication that it is appropriate.

On one of our first days in operation, before we were even positive where our television set would reside, I was informed of a video activity in progress. A staff member had brought in a videotape that was, I had no doubt, completely inappropriate. It was a 1940s-vintage, grade B, black-and-white detective drama, with no recognizable stars.

131

I had never heard of it before and don't now recall the title. I strolled to the area in question to see just how badly the show had fared.

All current residents (a handful, at that point) were watching the television attentively. So was the staff member who had supplied the film. Half an hour later, with staff trading off time with the tube, no one had left the room (although several individuals were sound asleep). Folks will, by and large, watch almost anything if a staff member or volunteer is watching with them. Even staff in-service training videos can make for rapt, "captive" viewing.

In selecting videotapes, do not necessarily discount staff interests. Overall, we're likely to get more mileage from videos, both commercial and homemade, than from TV shows. Here is a listing of some effective and appropriate videos. (Note: Films are often shown in half-hour segments ("chapters") or repeatedly, in traditional theater style.)

Newish Movies

- *Three Men and a Baby*
- *ET*
- *Coal Miner's Daughter*
- *Sweet Dreams*
- *That's Dancing*
- *That's Entertainment I & II*
- *The Homecoming* (and other Waltons videos)
- *Oliver*
- *Benjie*
- *The Black Stallion*
- *Beauty and the Beast*
- *Home Alone*

Oldish Movies

- *The African Queen*
- *Babes in Arms*
- *Bringing Up Baby*
- *Captain January*
- *Carousel*

- *Gone with the Wind*
- *The Incredible Journey*
- *The King and I*
- *Singin' in the Rain*
- *The Sound of Music*
- *Summer Stock*
- *The Wizard of Oz*
- *This Is the Army*

Other Videos

- Any episode of *I Love Lucy*
- Almost any episode of *Golden Girls*
- Lawrence Welk (especially with the "classic" cast; available from catalog 12)
- *Little House on the Prairie* videos
- Irving Berlin tapes. (Until his death, there were various all-star salutes to Mr. Berlin. These, like his music, have magical qualities.)
- Most any nature show
- *Barnyard Babies, Babies of the Home,* etc.
- *Whitetail Deer: Their Real World, Bear Babies,* etc. (Wild Life Unlimited Foundation, P.O. Box 312, Vesper, Wisconsin 54489)
- *Acadia* (various other titles: *Portraits of National Parks,* American Visions Services, Film and Video Center)
- Collections of "classic" comedies (Keystone Cops, Laurel and Hardy, etc.)

• A Few Good Video Catalogs (Films, TV Shows)

The Video Catalog
   P.O. Box 64267
   St. Paul, MN 55164-0428

Critics Choice Video
   P.O. Box 749
   Itasca, IL 60143-0749

Time Warner Viewer's Edge
   P.O. Box 3925
   Milford, CT 06460

Captain Bijou (A great source of all sorts of memorabilia)
   P.O. Box 87
   Toney, AL 35773-008

Barnes & Noble
   126 5th Ave.
   New York, NY 10011

• Three TV Tales •

Hank had been living alone. He was very fond of a local female newscaster. Each evening, at home, he would prepare cocktails and a meal for her and wait for the newscast. When she appeared, he proceeded to have his own drink (or drinks) and to grow enraged that she played "hard to get" and refused to join him.

Hank's family had assumed that he was simply growing delusional. After his admission to the A.C.C., the staff took care that, if a newscast was on, it was not Hank's "friend." Hank really enjoyed watching television and was not upset by appropriate programing.

One evening, nearly a year later, that particular channel was switched on and he caught sight of the same newscaster, his "old flame." He refused to let anyone near the television and grew upset (even lacking the cocktails).

During the Persian Gulf crisis and war, there was some curiosity about our handling of the situation.

We tried to avoid bringing it up. Did we try to shield our folks from that "reality"? To an extent, yes. We answered questions honestly but made no mention of it otherwise. In fact, many of the details of the situation were not likely to make much impression on folks with dementia: a war? about what—oil? where? who? The concept of a war, though, and of half a million American troops being committed overseas, was potentially traumatic.

We largely controlled the televiewing by programing the old-movie stations and using videotapes. An occasional news bulletin was, nonetheless, inevitable. One resident did begin to speak of "listening to the president," but most folks remained oblivious to it.

There was only one traumatic incident during the whole period. One gentleman suddenly grew frantic, watching the television, crying out, "Oh, no. Oh, God, this is awful: we're at war! We've been attacked!"

The television, however, was tuned to a movie channel. An old newsreel was airing and it showed Roosevelt giving his "Day of Infamy" speech.

A very popular Saturday morning activity is not unfamiliar in many "normal" households: watching television. I recently observed this pastime. A fairly large group was watching TV. They were very attentive and responsive. Indeed, their responsiveness showed a marked familiarity with the specific program.

I had occasionally heard one resident, Donna, refer to seeing "big" or "large" men on Saturdays. I had forgotten to follow this up by asking the staff who she might have meant: weekend visitors? maintenance workers? (Donna does, often, retain memory traces of specific incidents and people, though she tends to use very indirect or oblique words to describe them.)

That morning, watching folks watch TV, I learned who the "big men" on Saturday were. Grinning, Donna pointed toward the screen and said, "There: we're watching those big men." The program was professional wrestling. (I watched for any signs of disturbance at the "violence," such as the Three Stooges can trigger in some individuals, but saw none. Staff members assured me that they had never noticed anyone agitated by wrestling. Evidently, even with dementia, no one took the show as anything other than plain entertainment.

·: 9 :·

Cooking

There can be three types of food-related activity programs: those in which we talk about food, those in which we prepare food, and those in which we eat food. Although many (ideal) activities combine all three, this chapter deals with only the last two.

• Foods We Prepare •

The range of food-preparation tasks provides many examples of dementia-appropriate activity. These tasks tend to be familiar and well rehearsed (cutting, chopping, peeling, stirring, spreading), service-oriented (preparing food for others), and quickly gratifying (sampling while working, and eating the proceeds shortly after preparation). Most of the therapeutic benefits of traditional arts and crafts occur naturally in food preparation: at a "successful," appropriate, cognitive level, and in a meaningful context. A dementia-appropriate approach reverses our normal quest for shortcuts.

Coleslaw provides a model food-preparation activity. It is excellent task occupation for individuals at various cognitive levels. Slaw for fifty takes a lot of chopping, slicing, grating, etc. The opposite of a dementia-appropriate activity is to make coleslaw using a food processor.

We maintain an assortment of rather dull paring knives in a locked drawer in our kitchen. (Contrary to the old adage, these dull blades do not cut deepest. Luckily, we have never had a cut finger.) One astute individual did complain about the poor quality of our knives. We finally bought a sharpener and kept one sharp knife reserved for her. A "helper" usually provides a final, finer chopping, using a big butcher knife.

Dementia-appropriate cooking need not be done "from scratch." Rather, it should begin where tasks requiring measuring end. Measuring is well beyond the cognitive abilities of most people with dementia and should be bypassed. The measuring process can also be fairly time-consuming and makes for a less than enthralling spectator sport. To this end, prepared mixes are very useful. We usually start with prepared batter, either from a mix or from our dietary department.

This chapter does not offer actual recipes. The best recipes for any given program are likely to come from within its own "family." Many "kids' cooking" ideas are well suited for people with dementia or for mixed groups.

• Foods We Share •

Meals or snacks have various purposes. These can include extra nutrition (finger food, "fun" food, or snacks), seasonal pertinence (leftover sandwiches the day after Thanksgiving), or regional variations in "nostalgic" foods (grits). Above all, eating activities lend themselves to choice. Simple decision-making is often helped by the visual nature of the foods. Some examples follow of meals or snacks that need not involve much preparation by residents (not including items mentioned as specific discussion topics).

- Ice cream (cones, floats, sundaes, etc.).
  Making ice cream is a traditional favorite with groups of all ages and in most settings, though it is neither quick nor easy if done with a crank-type maker. It can certainly make for a shared, "focus" activity.
- Pizza.
  The advantages of pizza include its being finger food, red in color, and fairly nutritious. Disadvantages include the fact that it is an unfamiliar food for many elderly eaters. Eating with one's fingers is not something that everyone is comfortable with (at least, in public).

- Cookouts/Barbecues.
  Besides being seasonably appropriate, these can be good fol-
  low-up to a discussion of, say, hot dogs.
- Hot dogs (or sausages) with toppings.
- Submarine sandwiches (heroes, dagwoods, etc.).
  These provide a lot of choice and interest if the ingredients are
  spread out on platters, more or less deli-style. This arranging
  can be an engaging task in itself. Tongs are offered on the
  platters, but most of the actual assembling may be done by
  staff members or volunteers standing behind the serving ta-
  ble. (As the food is somewhat exposed while serving, and as
  flies tend to appear, we discontinue these meals during the
  summer months.)
- "Greasy spoon/Truck stop" breakfast.
  We offer choices of eggs, meats, home fries, etc., served in appropriate decor and costume.
- Blueberry pancake breakfast.
- "Grange suppers" (Baked Bean/Casserole/Hot Dish/Covered
  Dish Suppers).
- Doughnuts or doughnut holes, in variety.
  A uniquely sociable snack.
- Boiled lobster or steamed crabs.
  This is fine, make-work finger food. Fairly well rehearsed by
  many, the art of eating a whole lobster or crab is relatively
  new. Alternatives include lobster roll and seafood salad,
  which require a lot of preparatory work.

• A Baker's Dozen of Good Food Activities •

1. Picnic Lunch for Fifty
   We usually make three sandwich choices on white and dark
   bread. We have invariably found that more than three choices
   is overwhelming to almost everyone. Our favorite is peanut
   butter and jelly, though egg salad offers more basic work in
   the making. Sandwiches work best when served with finger
   foods such as potato chips, sliced cucumbers, and pickles. Po-

tato salad makes excellent work, but mixing fork food with finger food can be confusing to some.

2. Thumbprint Cookies

A staple of "kids' cooking," this is a high-success activity. Any easy-to-make or prepared recipe is usable, as long as it can be "balled." We usually find sugar cookie dough to be preferable. We have good success with the dough our kitchen prepares. We've found, though, that commercially prepared (frozen) dough tends to yield a stonelike cookie.

The tasks involved are quite basic; even the thumbprinting task itself is of midlevel difficulty. What actually goes into the print can vary widely. Cherries are easy to work with, easy to see, readily available, and available in colors (red and green) that lend themselves to many seasonal themes.

A variation is to bake the cookies in petit four tins. The tins themselves can add a bit of structure to the process. Also, if the filling is something like strawberry jam or blueberry sauce, the tins help control overflow.

3. Most other cookies—especially if prepared with cookie cutters.

4. Absolute Desperation Cookies for High Tea

Take one box of vanilla wafer cookies. Arrange on a work sheet. Decorate with frosting (spread or squirted on). Arrange on a tray, and serve with panache.

5. Birthday and/or Tea Cupcakes

A birthday cake can provide occupation for one or two folks, but cupcakes can involve almost any number. Cupcakes using petit four tins provide even more work. (When it comes to actually eating them, one can have two or even three and scarcely equal a "real" cupcake.)

Some tasks, such as actually filling the cups, are fairly demanding. Decorating the cooked products is, naturally, a very inexact science. Spreading plain frosting is a basic task; manipulating a "squirt" tube can be more demanding, although very enjoyable.

Cupcakes can easily be frozen for spur-of-the-moment decorating (or making work).

We usually keep extra boxes of frosting mix on hand. It is cheap and you just add water. Stirring it, perhaps with some food coloring added, can be very involving and tension-releasing. It can also provide an alternative, basic task during a group work session (such as sandwich making).

6. Apple Pie

Can't be beat. Use your own, or anyone else's, recipe. Making the crust may not be a good dementia-appropriate activity; consider using prepared crusts.

7. Any Other Apple Stuff

Anything using apples makes excellent work. To many cooks, the act of coring apples is a fairly automatic task. Apples are among the most "reminiscent" foods.

8. Potato Salad (or coleslaw)

9. Fruit Salad (avoiding kiwi fruit)

10. Soup

Making soup is a good weekend activity. It takes a good deal of work, cooks for a long time, smells great while cooking, and has many traditional aspects: few things are homier than homemade soup and sandwiches. The process can begin early Saturday, especially if there is a chicken to be cooked and picked apart. Chicken soup makes a lot of work (and is great during cold and flu season). Pea soup is also popular.

We have found that making sandwiches along with the soup, in addition to Sunday religious activities, family visits, and refreshments for Sunday afternoon social activity, is a bit much. It has worked well when our kitchen provided grilled cheese sandwiches to accompany the soup.

11. Popcorn Balls

12. Gingerbread (with or without whipped cream)

Few foods have a more evocative taste than gingerbread. Hand-whipping the cream is great busywork.

13. Old-fashioned Venison Mincemeat

This is an ideal dementia-appropriate activity, although not all the required ingredients are easily obtained. It lends a lot of reminiscence value as well, and the aroma of the long cooking is intoxicating.

The key ingredient is the neck of at least one deer. The neck meat is very stringy and perfect for a variety of hands to "pick." Any good recipe should come with directions.

Of course, any item such as mincemeat or pickles should be eaten immediately, in accordance with state health regulations. That is not to say that homemade delicacies—mincemeat and pickles, for example—could not be brought from private homes for special events, such as Thanksgiving dinner.

• Some Ideas That Didn't Work •

The working tenet, "Nothing ventured, nothing gained," is at its most dangerous around food (especially meals). Over the years, we have tried many food-related ideas. There follow a few that we have either not repeated or have finally given up on.

- Homemade bread
  (Although it can be a wonderful task, the more often the better, in a private home.)
- Tacos
  The tacos were even soft-shelled, more like burritos, but our folks had never seen the like and simply stared at them. Peanut butter and jelly sandwiches saved the day.
- Pigs in blankets
  They seemed like a good idea, but they were very difficult to make and too craftlike. Then, no one knew what they were. The hot dogs hidden inside went unnoticed and uneaten. The trusty peanut butter and jelly sandwiches and a big afternoon snack saved that day, too!
- Most oriental foods
- Gelatin "jiggler" things (using cookie cutters)
  These are a bit hard to handle in the making, and they tend not to look like food when done.

• A Recipe for Reliably Clean Hands •

A frequent obstacle to dementia-appropriate cooking concerns hygiene—primarily folks' hands. Individuals often will reply, "Oh, I just washed my hands," or, indignantly, "I keep my hands clean!" Further, hand-washing techniques sometimes leave a bit to be desired.

The key is dishwashing liquid. Advertising claims aside, Dawn is the brand environmentalists use for cleaning oil off birds after an oil spill: it cuts grease (i.e., cleans) better than other brands.

Folks rarely object to having a bit of liquid gently poured, lotionlike, onto their hands (especially if everyone else is doing it). Once the liquid is applied, vigorous, careful hand-washing is the nearly automatic result.

If individuals refuse to wash their hands (or to "rewash," having left the kitchen and returned), then their active involvement in the work might be limited or redirected.

·: 10 :·

Gardening

The therapeutic uses of horticulture, in its myriad aspects, are ancient and effective, adaptable, and almost limitless. Ardent gardeners typically spend endless hours simply strolling, slowly and savoringly, through their gardens, alone or with chosen friends. The recreational and/or therapeutic uses of gardening range far beyond active soil cultivation, planting, and weeding. Many people have some long-standing, and long-enjoyed, involvement with gardening.

At the A.C.C. the garden is a focal point of the environment. The design of the actual garden area combines different types of gardens (raised-bed planters, specialized plantings) with dementia-specific adaptations.

Simply getting outdoors is at the most basic level of therapy. Most folks in the early to middle stages of dementia, and sometimes even beyond, still love and crave getting outside. They have not developed that hot-house syndrome, endemic in nursing homes, in which no hot summer day is warm enough for them to tolerate the great out-of-doors. Nonetheless, shade should be a built-in feature of any enjoyable garden. Older folks should always have access to sunglasses and hats, whether their own or communal.

The design of the central garden encourages self-guided walking. The garden path is a hundred-foot oval, and the outer edge of the perennial planting is high enough to block the lines of sight. Thus, every lap around tends to be the "first" time. Every time an individual strolls around and sees the cheery daffodils, or admires the elegant iris, or sniffs the perfumed stocks, the experience registers as a new discovery. The path also provides an ideal setting for group walks.

The grounds of the A.C.C. also afford the enjoyment of nature. Around the building is a tranquil space of lawn, meadow, trees, and small areas of woods. Surrounded by a reasonably unobtrusive fence ("to keep the wild animals out"), the grounds promote quiet and relatively secure strolling.

Actual work on the garden and grounds is more problematical, but some of the classic and useful dementia activities involve grounds maintenance. Such chores include raking leaves and grass clippings and sweeping and raking walkways. An old push-mower continues to invite independent use "in season." A wheelbarrow is also put to frequent, and sometimes rather surprising, use. Stacks of firewood tend to be moved and restacked.

A useful "long cut" garden chore is a bucket brigade. What could be accomplished in little time with a hose or sprinkler can readily involve several individuals, all busy and useful, watering flowers and vegetables with plastic watering cans. The "foreperson" simply keeps the watering cans filled (and perhaps takes the hose around later, unseen, to ensure a deep watering for all needy areas). This task provides some exercise (especially if the watering cans are more than half full), has little chance of failure, and is quite self-cuing. Rarely, if ever, has anyone asked, "Why not just use the hose?" "White lie" ploys are easy to imagine: "The hose won't reach," "These beds need that personal touch," "This way everybody can lend a hand."

Much actual work depends on individual cognitive levels. Soil preparation, with hand tools, spades, etc., is a task that many can undertake successfully and with perseverance.

The skills involved in planting either seeds or seedlings may well erode fairly early in dementia. It is not uncommon for even experienced gardeners, now coping with dementia, to plant the marigold upside down, to try to eat the petunia, to bury the flat of alyssum intact. Using step-by-step, hand-over-hand cuing, however—and a bit of sleight-of-hand—folks can, on a one-to-one basis, be involved in a very satisfying task.

Planting bulbs is more likely to be feasible than planting seeds. When folks are able to plant, the work plan naturally needs to be very flexible.

Practiced gardeners can often dead-head, or pinch off dead blossoms, with minimal cuing. This is not only time-consuming but also quite necessary work for many annuals.

The task of weeding is likewise within the abilities of some folks, even when the ability to discriminate between weed and flower is not (aside from the fact that one gardener's weed may well be another's flower!). Annuals are, of course, easily replaced, and after June begin to plummet in price. (By midsummer, some hardware stores, markets, and greenhouses may be glad to donate replacement annuals, rather than continue to water them.)

Many summer activity programs can have their roots in the garden. Seasonal produce, whether homegrown or not, can provide discussion, work, and socialization in the eating. Herbs can also have thematic connections. For example, a discussion of "home remedies" could include a garden tour of medicinal herbs. Flowers can be cut as a group project and arranged—a nice alternative to bouquets donated from funeral homes. They could be picked individually, stuck into button-holes, or given to someone else. Varieties of everlastings, if dried, will last all winter.

The use of scented plants is one of the oldest aspects of horticulture in general, and of horticultural therapy in particular. Some loss of smell and taste may be inevitable with the aging process, and these losses may or may not be more severe with dementia. Most folks, though, still love the acts of smelling and tasting (even if the ability to discriminate between, say, two scents, is lost). With individuals fairly well along in the disease, some caution should be exercised, as an invitation to smell will trigger a response to eat.

• "Good Scents" Annuals •

In the following list, plants marked with a double asterisk (**) reseed themselves readily; those marked with a single asterisk (*) may be hard to find commercially, although the seed can easily be ordered and grown.

- (White) Sweet alyssum**
- Four-o'clocks (*Mirabilis*) (These bloom in the early evening and close up in the morning.)
- Heliotrope*
- Marigold

- Mignonette* (A Victorian favorite; may have lost some scent over the years, but is still well worth the sniffing; notably unshowy as flowers go.)
- *Nicotiana alta** and *N. sylvestris** (Woodland tobacco) (Unlike most varieties of Nicotiana, which no longer have much scent, even at night, these two are powerful.)
- Petunia (Deep purple/blue varieties.)
- "Red rocket" snapdragon
- Sweet pea
- Stock
- Sweet sultan* (*Centaura imperialis*) (Some commercial seed is not true and will blossom into plain bachelor's buttons.)
- Scented geranium. (A special case: annual or herb? house plant or garden flower? In any case, it can thrive if treated like an annual. While the flowers are minimal, at least compared to their vibrant namesakes, the foliage is wonderfully fragrant. The old-fashioned rose geranium will be familiar to many folks. While many newer varieties are cultivated with foliage and/or flowers in mind, many of the various scented types— lemon, lime, ginger, apple, nutmeg, coconut, etc.—are fascinating to the curious nose.)
- Note: *Datura* (Jimsonweed), sometimes listed as a fragrant annual, is a potentially lethal hallucinogenic, even in small doses. It is extremely poisonous and should be identified and treated as such if allowed to remain on facility grounds.

• "Good Scents" Perennials •

Those marked with an asterisk (*) may be tricky to find. None of the following is known to be dangerous if eaten.

- Bee balm (*Monarda*)
- Perennial varieties of dianthus, or pinks (In some zones, best treated as annuals.)
- Gas plant (*Dictamnus*)*
- (Garden) Heliotrope (*Valerianella officinallis*)
- Jacob's ladder

- Plantain lily (*Hosta grandiflora*)
- Roses (!)
- Sweet rocket (*Hesperis matronalis*)
- Sweet fern (*Comptonia asplinifolia*).* (Not usually thought of as a plant to be cultivated—in other words, a weed.) A "volunteer" appeared in a very convenient spot in our perennial bed a few years ago. It has developed into a lush, compact, drought- and insect-resistant shrub. Its distinctive, wild, and definitely sweet scent pervades the whole area, and even the indoors, if the windows are open.

• Culinary Herbs •

A primary use of culinary herbs is for scent. However, many salt-free kitchens find themselves revolutionized by a little "herbal therapy" (including garlic and—with discretion—hot peppers). All can be freely sampled for scent and/or (with the exception of lavender) taste.

As our herbs are all located in planters, to be readily seen, touched, and sniffed, none is reliably hardy.

Annual:

- Anise
- Basil (Green or purple, plain or ruffled; such new variations as lemon and licorice basil are a bit baffling to folks with dementia.)
- Coriander (Its rank scent is noxious to some, but is certainly noticeable.)
- Dill (A traditional staple! Reseeds freely.)
- Lemon verbena
- Parsley

Perennial:

- Lavender
- Lemon balm
- Mints in variety (while very hardy, mint tends to cross-pollinate

or to revest to an earlier strain. Will also take over any bed in which it is planted.)

- Rosemary
- Sage
- Thyme in variety (Traditionally used in walkways, among many other ways.)

• Medicinal Herbs •

Most herbs have some medicinal use. The following are potentially interesting and/or useful to grow.

A really effective cough cure:

- Horehound
- Hyssop
- Pennyroyal (mint)
- Spearmint and peppermint

The first two have very distinctive scents and rather unpleasant tastes. Properly picked and dried, however, these two ingredients, combined in a tea or decoction with (at least) equal parts of peppermint and spearmint, make a very effective expectorant. Hyssop also is a very attractive flowering shrub and lasts quite a while as a dried flower. Folks will recall pennyroyal as a traditional cure-all, found wild.

Herbs for mental processes:

Certain herbs have historically been associated with improving mentation, in terms of both alertness and overall memory. These include:

- Coltsfoot (in liquid preparation)
- Lavender (in a potpourri or sachet)
- Lemon balm (in liquid preparation)
- Peppermint (in a dry mix or a decoction)
- Rosemary (in liquid preparation)

A nontraditional herb now universally recommended for enhancing memory is gotu kola.

Herbs for relaxation:

Some herbs have been traditionally associated with relieving anxiety. These, as teas, include:

- Catnip
- Chamomile
- Hops
- Lavender
- Lemon balm

• Everlastings •

The number of plant materials that can be dried and used in arrangements and crafts is virtually endless. The following list contains a few varieties that are easily obtained (either as seed or as seedling), grown, gathered, dried, and used.

Drying these simply consists in first picking them just before they fully open (preferably mid- to late morning, when the dew has dried). With the leaves gently stripped off, the flowers can simply be hung upside down in a dry, nonsunny place for a week or two. Once dry, the flowers can be arranged on their own stems, impaled on floral wire, or used in whatever way is desired.

Annual:

- Acroclinium
- Helicrysum (Strawflowers)
- Statice (in its wide range of colors)
- Xeranthemum

Perennial:

- Baby's breath (*Gypsophila*)
- Globe amaranth (*Gomphrena*)
- Sea lavender (*Limomium*)
- Yarrow (*Achillea*) (Note: should be planted with discretion—for example, in containers—as it is very invasive.)

• A Few Good Things to Have Growing Here and There All Summer Long •

Flowers

- Coleus (Another item that few self-respecting landscapers would ever use, but colorful, easy, and always attention-grabbing. Best grown away from direct sunlight.)
- Cosmos (Beautiful, showy flowers that bloom for a long time; re-seed themselves reliably. They tend to bend in the wind, so they do best in sheltered locations, as against a wall. No scent, but they press nicely.)
- Portulaca (One of the most cheerful flowers; loves dry conditions. It will reseed in large numbers, though the flowers become more single, growing more "unhybridized" each year—it reverts to purslane, its edible wild form. A benefit of growing portulaca is that it creates a lot of work: the numerous flowers must be dead-headed (pinched off) frequently, as the blossoms live for only two days. If the dead flowers are not pinched off, the plant will look positively ratty and will stop flowering.)
- Salpiglossis (Showy and interesting; smallish, petunialike flowers with vivid stripes of orange, yellow, blue, etc.)

Plant

- Sensitive plant (*Mimosa pudica*). (Often grown indoors. Looks like a small fern; the leaves curl up and stems collapse temporarily when touched.)

Vegetables

The first five are fast-growing varieties that thrive in containers as well as in a normal garden spot. The fast-growing varieties of container vegetables—especially tomatoes and cucumbers—are widely adaptable.

- Chives (and garlic chives)
- "Tokyo cross" turnip greens
- "Little finger" carrots

- French breakfast radish (Doesn't turn "hot.")
- Tiny Tim (cherry) or Sweet 100 tomatoes
- Purple beans (These are available under a variety of names, but all are purple on the outside as they grow. When cooked, they turn green and taste like any "normal" string bean.)
- Squash (Several members of the squash family can be grown for interest. These include gourds, in any of the endless shapes and colors; spaghetti squash, a fairly recent novelty, which can create an interesting taste test; and even zucchini, which is still novel to many older people.)

·: 11 :·

Pets

Most homes have much-loved stories about pets and other animals. Residential care facilities, regardless of level, are usually no exception. Animals can have a magical effect on people of all varieties, including varying disabilities and ages. The growth and value of visiting-pet programs in various settings have been well publicized.

Pets are, in many ways, like children in terms of their appeal—their nearly automatic ability to produce smiles and an air of optimism. Pets are also like children in that, at least for individuals and populations with dementia, they are most effective in small numbers for limited periods of time—in the proverbial small doses.

We usually think of "therapeutic" pets as being dogs and cats. They are generally easier to manage and more familiar to individuals. Dogs and cats are laden with reminiscing value. They are also readily available. The numbers of other creatures effective on an in-house visiting basis, however, is almost unlimited. Somewhat unusual examples include ferrets, lambs, pigs, turkeys, geese, rabbits, and turtles.

Any animal that has made guest appearances in schools is likely to work well elsewhere. A visiting animal is even more likely to be effective if paired with its offspring. Obvious concerns regarding individual animals include temperament (geese are not always the most gregarious creatures and hyperactive dogs are agitating), cleanliness/hygiene (no animals would be preferable to soiled or unhealthy ones), practicality (a 300-pound hog would be difficult to accommodate in some settings), and pertinent public health or state regulations. Some care should be exercised with animals that might have "shock value." Rats and snakes jump to mind as potentially provocative pet therapy participants.

If outdoor space is available, then the ante is upped a bit. Donkeys, horses, sheep, and llamas have all been used as effective visitors.

There is nothing new about animals living in residential facilities. Cats, birds, and fish are nearly universal examples. Not all cats are suited for congregate living, but many adapt extremely well. Parakeets, canaries, and other birds are easily maintained and can be cheerful additions. The calming, distracting aspects of watching tropical fish are not limited to the dentist's office.

All animals, however, can present their own challenges.

The A.C.C. was originally envisioned as having a variety of pets in residence. One early thought was to include a border collie or other herding breed in hopes of combining companionship with protectiveness. But it was decided that the vigor with which such dogs work to keep their charges "at home" might be dangerous to the residents. Some working breeds or individual dogs are prone to high energy levels, if not plain nervousness, especially if not in true working settings.

The first nonhuman resident at the A.C.C. was Sootie, a year-old, neutered female cat. Her name stemmed from smudges of gray on her forehead. She was otherwise completely white. Sootie was a known quantity in terms of temperament; she had literally grown up in a visiting-pet therapy program. When the A.C.C. opened, Sootie was slightly overdue for "graduation," and moved in. She adjusted immediately and to the delight of all cat-lovers.

The question of a residential dog was unresolved as our opening date approached. Then, at the eleventh hour, a solution appeared. The National Seeing Eye Foundation wished to find placement for a special dog. His name was Pal.

Every dog is the best dog in the world. Pal may, in many ways, have in fact been the world's best dog. He was eight years old, mostly black Lab, with a touch of something else. He had been a Seeing Eye dog for about six years. His home had been in one of the world's largest cities; he had traveled the world. Then his master regained his sight and was not able to retain Pal. A dog of eight was deemed too old to retrain; hence the urgency for placement.

Pal came to the A.C.C. for visits, during which it appeared clear that he was the perfect resident pet. A month after it opened, Pal came to live at the A.C.C. No dog could have come to his new life with more conscientiousness, intelligence, sensitivity, and sweetness. He became an instant fixture.

By and by, a parakeet named Sarah Lee needed a home. She was moved in on a trial basis. One major concern was the effect of the bird's singing on folks: would it be cheering or uniquely annoying? It was the former; she stayed. (Fortunately, the state had relaxed an earlier prohibition against having birds living in residential health-care facilities.) The only problem with Sarah Lee came when her melodic trilling created the idea in certain individuals that she was hungry and/or thirsty. Typically, this is not a problem but a challenge, usually amenable to redirection and reassurance.

Another potential challenge with animals in residence is possessiveness. It is true that a cat is usually on the wrong side of the door, but with multiple "owners," the problem is compounded.

For two years our only cat problems were of the usual dead rodent/live snake variety. Sootie helped the possessiveness situation considerably by carefully dividing her time, sleeping on different beds and in different laps in a fairly set routine. The problem developed, though, with a specific new resident, Oscar. This very independent, strong-willed man rapidly identified Sootie as his own (despite the fact that he had never owned a white cat). He grew assaultive to anyone who went near Sootie. Before long, he was restraining the cat in dresser drawers and barricading his room to keep the cat in and others out.

Oscar's handling of the cat was also less than gentle—a potential problem for both Sootie, who was several times rescued from what appeared to be imminent danger, and Oscar. Even this patient, gentle creature would presumably have her limits of "manhandling." Meanwhile, the eight or nine other "owners" of the cat grew increasingly possessive in turn. Altercations over ownership, questions of in-or-out ("That's *my* cat and she wants to go out"; "It is not, it's *my* cat and I want him in!"), etc., grew increasingly frequent.

A solution was suggested: get a black cat. That might at least defuse the ownership "wars." A local shelter was glad to provide an adult, neutered, black female cat: Rebecca. She did, in fact, adjust nicely, both with the residents and, after a bit of territorial squabbling, with Sootie. The effect was quickly apparent. All eight or nine cat owners were now the proud owners of two cats: one white and one black. One lady began referring to her "gray" cat.

Oscar, however, grew, if anything, even more possessive of Sootie.

Shortly afterward, a temporary home was found for Sootie, in a nearby residential facility. When Oscar ultimately left us to move to a nursing home closer to his family, Sootie returned, settling in as if she had never left. One of her former "owners," a resident who spent a great deal of time in her room, observed, with tears in her eyes: "My white cat has finally come home to me."

Not long afterward, another cat was rumored to need a home. This was a neutered, yellow-and-white male, received on Christmas morning by a delighted little girl. Unfortunately, her father quickly discovered a hitherto unknown allergy to cats. Snickers was said to have a good disposition and seemed to offer a good color contrast. He moved in for a trial period, quickly becoming a family member more or less accepted by Sootie and Rebecca.

Pal, however, was not as happy. After a year or so, he grew noticeably lethargic, generally acting sad. He increasingly avoided group situations, seeking several specific staff members to accompany on a one-to-one basis. He actually began to avoid "jobs" that he had previously accepted, such as joining both indoor and outdoor walks.

Two staff members began to take Pal home for occasional weekends. The difference in the dog was dramatic. In the private homes, he was more alert, active, downright playful. However, he grew a bit more distraught every time he came back "home" to the center. The "R & R" weekends became more frequent, and there was no carryover in his attitude after returning to the A.C.C.

After a bit less than two years, Pal finally went to live at one of his weekend homes. It is a multigenerational home, and Pal has been a very happy, valued, and much-loved member of the family ever since.

This pattern has recurred with many other dogs in many residential situations. The right dog can be a valuable addition to any program, but the animal needs to be able to leave its "work" at night. Dogs living in residential situations tend, very simply, to grow depressed. Lethargy and social withdrawal (such as with Pal) are common. Also common, though not present with Pal, are loss of appetite and skin conditions.

Recently, Rebecca, by now eight years old, went to live with a staff member as well. She had been growing a bit testy with the residents and had scratched one person in an (understandable) effort to jump down. She had also been increasingly untidy in her habits. She, too, is doing well now.

We periodically discuss setting up an aquarium. These discussions are usually derailed by questions of maintenance and finding a safe place for it. It's not hard to picture a freestanding aquarium being toppled over by someone busily attempting to do only-she-knows-what to it. Anyone who has ever experienced a hundred-gallon aquarium in a health-care facility springing a leak for no apparent reason will hesitate to risk dealing with a second. (A videotape of tropical fish has recently been found notably uninteresting to our folks. A soundtrack may help.)

Often, individuals with dementia do not perceive that certain, realistic stuffed animals are inanimate. They will often discuss them when passing by, speak to them, even pat them. When Sootie went to live elsewhere, one woman in particular, Mildred, grieved her loss. She was somewhat consoled by a stuffed white cat. Although the bond between human and stuffed animal is a diluted version of the real thing, it is still significant.

• Bears •

Teddy Bears are probably the most common stuffed animals. A number of "talking" bears and other creatures are now available. These feature sound devices, whether a simple cassette playing tapes or a tape recorder for recording and repeating what is said to it. Years ago I had a plush Christmas Moose vanish which, when its red, lighted "heart" was pressed, would play a medley of Christmas songs. The "Spinosa" bear, for instance (from catalog 12), is becoming common from children's day-care centers to nursing homes to hospital emergency rooms. Each bear comes equipped with a set of tapes. These are designed to be relaxing/reassuring programs, using spoken messages and original songs. When used with dementia-appropriate tapes, these can be quite effective.

One lady, Ina, came to us for a week of respite care equipped with a cassette tape of her daughter's and granddaughters' voices. Tried in a "talking" bear, however, these personal messages, rather than being reassuring, tended to cause Ina to frantically search for her loved ones. But another individual, Juanita, is quite calmed by the same bear. She tends to become anxious after lunch; if given the bear in a quiet setting—usually a staff office—she will happily sit and listen to a tape of Tennessee Ernie Ford singing hymns from the bear (which she usually refers to as a "puppy"). She has actually learned that the "puppy" or "that man" will sing to her, although not how to turn it on. She typically sits very intently with the bear and the music. When the human companionship is gone, however passive it may have been, Juanita loses interest in the bear. She will sit alone, or "independently," under one condition only: if she actually falls asleep.

• A Special Tale •

Carlos had always had three main interests: his family, his job, and his cellar workshop. According to his son, he had always been busy: "If he wasn't working, he had to have a project going, usually three or four at a time." Carlos's wife commented that, after retiring, he "practically lived down cellar."

At the A.C.C., Carlos was not one to join group activities. He was also difficult to involve in one-to-one tasks, preferring usually to follow his own designs. He was, however, very energetic and very busy, usually after midnight. Unfortunately, his "projects" were sometimes disruptive: attempting to move chairs (occupied or otherwise) through solid walls, banging "panic bars" on emergency exits, disconnecting the television, and so on.

One staff member wondered if, given Carlos's history, a workbench might attract him; one was purchased and assembled. In fact, the workbench did appear to attract him; various male-oriented projects left to be "discovered" on it did help occupy him. But I was alarmed to notice that most mornings the workbench ended up cluttered with "cute" stuffed animals. The "manly" items left for Carlos were either buried or not even in sight; the workbench was being used as a catch-all for stuffed animals. I noticed this disturbing phenomenon a while before finally remembering to mention it, rather indignantly, to fellow staff members. I was kindly and patiently informed that the collections of stuffed animals were, in fact, Carlos' handiwork: that he spent hours each night quietly collecting every stuffed animal he could lay his hands on, arranging and rearranging them on his work bench, happily chatting with each and every one.

·: 12 :·

Spirituality

It is difficult to evaluate the spiritual needs of individuals with dementia. However, the rapt attentiveness of participants in dementia-appropriate worship services should be sufficient testimony to the value of structured worship. No single activity produces more pronounced and predictable effects of, in a word, peacefulness.

Some individuals will consistently choose not to participate in any religious activity; these tend to be the ones who do not participate in groups generally. Others may react catastrophically; these tend to be individuals with a history of aversion to religion. Some will vary from day to day, like the lady who was raised Catholic, shunned religious involvement through most of her adulthood, then became a Jehovah's Witness in late years. These differences must simply be accepted and adapted to, like any others.

Overall, religious activity should follow the basic principles of any dementia-appropriate activity. If volunteers are involved, then it is important that they use the same approaches and techniques as other volunteers (and staff). Formal services should be brief and simple—short on sermons, heavy on hymns. Scripture and prayers should be familiar and brief. Hymns should be the "old standards" (unless sung by children).

Denominational divisions, such as those within Christianity, tend to lose their importance as people grow older. To many nursing-home residents without dementia, the particular denomination of an individual Baptist minister will be less crucial than the fact that he or she is

Baptist. To others, the most important thing will simply be that this person is clergy. What is important, as our staff has said so many times, is "sharing the faith, not the doctrine." With dementia, these divisions—even those between Catholic and Protestant—can disappear altogether.

It is always important to bear in mind that, for the generations born closer to the beginning of this century than the end, a more or less formal religious upbringing was the norm. A church was for many children in those days what a television was to many baby boomers and their own offspring. It is not uncommon to see individuals with dementia growing more comfortable with the religion of their childhood. Some individuals avidly sing gospel songs who were never known to go to church in their adult years.

Some of the significance of religion in dementia has to do with nonverbal aspects. Visual symbols are powerful: a cross, a star of David, candles, a clerical collar, a yarmulkah. The rote gestures and responses, so well learned early and more or less often rehearsed over the years, tend to remain long into the disease: making the sign of the cross; accepting the host in Communion; obeying the command, "Let us pray"; repeating an "amen" and singing it at the end of a hymn; lighting Sabbath or Hanukkah candles; responses such as *Glory Be to God*; and the *Lord's Prayer*. These have an emotional effect on the participants. The act of going to church is very meaningful in itself. Individuals' involvement in their congregation of choice should certainly be maintained as long as possible, both at home and after admission to a residential facility.

• A Sort of Parable •

A quiet hymn can be the most powerfully reassuring, relaxing device of all.

One beautiful summer day, the usual midafternoon reading group convened. It had been a fairly calm day. As the reading progressed, the sky outside began to darken rapidly; the wind whipped into a gale. A thunderstorm appeared imminent. In what little was visible of the corridor beyond the doors, judging mostly from what shoes were passing and how rapid their pace was, I could see that anxiety was growing with the approaching storm and the plummeting barometer.

The behavior of one gentleman, prone to severe behavioral disturbances, was obviously escalating rapidly. Some days, he would join the reading group. Even if he stayed for only ten minutes, it would take the edge off whatever anxiety level he came in with. This was not one of those days. Staff members began to pair off with "escalating" individuals; their shoes joined those pacing past the door. One or two individuals were escorted in and joined us. Unfortunately, by this time it was three o'clock, time for the dreaded shift change.

I had already abandoned anything but singing. However, I had planned to save hymn-singing for later, after adjourning to the "big" room for a snack. Then, one individual began to bang on the doors. She came in, then immediately needed to leave. She then banged on the door again for admittance. I left the door open. Another lady strode in, rather frantic, describing a "big man" who was chasing her. A tall gentleman followed her in, to her annoyance, drawn by the singing.

The sound of someone "out there" calling for help was unmistakable. The twenty-five or so in the room were growing more than a little edgy. Then the storm burst. The rain pounded, roaring off the roof in torrents; the lightning looked as though it would burst the pine trees in the yard; the walls and floors of the building shook with every clap.

First we sang, *Amazing Grace,* then *Rock of Ages,* and then *When the Roll Is Called up Yonder.* We sang that, with all verses, again, and the effect, with the thunder and lightning as accompaniment, was almost giddy.

Suddenly, in plunged the highly agitated fellow, a staff member not far behind. He watched for a moment, began to sing in snippets, then sat down. He looked relieved; he stayed.

Fortunately, I had the *Reader's Digest Book of Inspirational Songs* on my lap. We sang hymns for twenty minutes. By that time, virtually every resident and adult day program participant in the building was in that room, clearly drawn by the sound of the hymns. I sat on a table; two men sat on the floor, having given their seats to women; one woman sat on a friend's lap. Staff members and a volunteer would pause, passing by, staring in with looks of surprise. They did not come in; there wasn't room for a cat in there.

At first, I had hoped that this would prove to be a brief, violent storm. That was, a staff member assured me, what the weather forecast called for. As we sang, the sky stopped growing darker; the rain seemed to lessen a bit; the thunder and lightning subsided slightly;

the air pressure was rising. We kept singing hymns, but they seemed more cheerful, optimistic, even triumphant.

With about the same speed that it had descended, the storm abated. When the sun came out again, the room lit up with smiles. As usual, we concluded with *May the Good Lord Bless and Keep You,* and adjourned. The group had lasted for over an hour and a half.

I don't remember what we had for a snack. Whatever it was, it had never tasted better. A quiet night was had by all.

Why did old gospel songs help calm and comfort that crowd, in the face of nature's fury, when nothing else, evidently, would? I would offer just one simple answer: because they were there. And I'll use gospel songs again, anytime.

Reality Orientation (R.O.)

Reality Orientation has long been the "traditional" approach to individuals confused about matters of person, place, and/or time. A basic system of interventions, it suggested a calm, respectful, matter-of-fact approach. It stressed the use of facts: where we are, what season and day it is, what the weather's like, and so on. Key aspects included simplified language, repetition, positive reinforcement, multi-sensory approaches and individualized care planning. Above all, teamwork and staff consistency were emphasized.

As sensibly taught, R.O. was neither persuasion nor teaching; honesty was valued but neither confrontation nor argument was a suggested technique. Structured R.O. group work or classes added important aspects of socialization and self-esteem: what could be termed "social security."

R.O. was fairly standardized long before "Alzheimer disease" was a familiar term. Its limitations owe more to our understanding about the special nature of A.D. and related dementias than to the methodology itself. A classic example is the well-meaning care giver attempting to help Mrs. X realize that if her mother were still alive, then the poor woman would be a hundred and forty years old; or, "Mrs. X, you were born in eighteen ninety-seven, and this is nineteen so-and-so: therefore, you must be ... " Folks with A.D. generally lack the cognitive ability for such logical, "if ... then," thinking. Such insight and most true learning are problematical at best. If Mr. Y is anxiously searching for his deceased wife, it is usually pointless (and cruel) to inform him that she is dead. The vital "reality," his inner reality, may simply be that he feels lonely or hungry.

Daily Activity Schedule

Time	One-on-One	Large Group (Core Activities)	Small Group
7:00 A.M.	Medication, whirl-pool, Continental breakfast		TV (old musicals, *Lucy*)
7:30	Walking outdoors, as needed (on-going)	Informal "fireside" group, coffee, etc.	"
8:00	Breakfast		
9:00	Nap (as needed), "quiet," toileting	Current events: daily paper, weather, etc.	Cleanup
9:30	"	Exercise group	Reading table
10:00	"	Coffee/juice break	Food preparation
10:30	Individual activities	Discussion topic of the day, guest musicians Musical interludes, guest musicians, etc.	Quiet time

11:30	All: Indoor/out-door walking, garden, toileting, dining-room/ lunch preparation		
12:00	———————————— Lunch ————————————		
1:00 P.M.	Nap in room, toileting	Quiet hour	Cleanup, brief reading, table activities
2:00	Table activities	TV, old movies	Table activities
2:30	"	Reading aloud	Setup for social activities
3:30		All: Tea, happy hour, ice cream social, dancing, entertainment	
4:00	Medication, personal care, etc.		Folding laundry
4:30	Toileting	Quiet singing, conversation	
5:30	———————————— Supper ————————————		
6:00	Whirlpool, toileting		Cleanup
6:30	Personal care, strolling, etc.	Evening reading	TV: sitcoms
7:30	"	Snacks	Snacks
8:00	"	Selected TV, video, films	Social groups, table activity

Remotivation Therapy

Remotivation Therapy is a simple and uniquely effective method of group therapy. It is as valuable and adaptable to the needs of any mentally challenged population as it was when first developed (by a volunteer) over thirty-five years ago. The object is to reach the "unwounded" areas of the individual's personality through an objective, nonthreatening social process. Each session, conducted by a trained leader, involves between six and fifteen participants and focuses on a specific topic. Topics are concrete, objective, and familiar in nature. Poetry, music, and other sensory aids are employed to gain and maintain group attention. Participants' thoughts, knowledge, and memories are drawn out by simple, structured questions relating to the topic. Feelings or opinions are not part of the process. The typical length of a session is roughly thirty minutes to an hour and the frequency, once or twice a week. With participants having A.D. or related dementia, groups may last for shorter periods and may be conducted more often.

The following is a very brief description of the five basic steps that make up a formal Remotivation session.

Step 1. The Climate of Acceptance

This is a "welcome"; each participant is greeted individually. The goal is to create a relaxed, cordial, and nonthreatening milieu.

Step 2. A Bridge to Reality

The topic is introduced. "Bounce Questions," simple, leading questions, are often used to inductively suggest the topic. A poem or song is typically used as well. Classic topics include animals, flowers, vegetables, foods and beverages, automobiles, school days, etc.: the more objective and specific, the better.

Step 3. Sharing the World We Live In

Specially selected questions are used to develop the topic and to invite individual contributions. Props related to the topic, ranging from simple pictures to manipulative objects, are often used. If the topic is "dogs," for example, the discussion aids could range from pictures to plastic models to a canine "guest."

Step 4. Appreciating the Work of the World

The original intent here was to engage participants in discussing and reminiscing about work: their own and others'. This step could also include more active involvement: eating apples or making applesauce, for example.

Step 5. The Climate of Appreciation

The session concludes with the leader summarizing aspects of the sessions, acknowledging individual contributions or responses, and appreciating each participants' involvement. There may also be some mention or development of the next session.

While Remotivation Therapy can be effectively practiced by nonprofessional caregivers, group leaders should receive formal training in the technique. Principles and methods of Remotivation often underlie and inform the practice of many therapists, whether or not they are conducting specific Remotivation Groups. The five basic steps and overall approach become second nature.

Remotivation training is easily available in most states. Questions regarding training availability may be directed to:

National Remotivation Therapy Organization Inc.
P.O. Box 361
Andover, MA 01810

Good Catalogs

The catalogs listed here are generally free of charge, and the materials they carry tend to be reasonably sturdy. Many items are carried by more than one catalog. And many items can be adapted or made "at home" for less than the amount charged in the specific catalogs.

This is more a list of sources for specific items than a comprehensive list of dementia resources. The titles are arranged alphabetically and are numbered only for the sake of reference.

1. AdaptABILITY
   (Designs for Independent Living)
       P.O. Box 515
       Colchester, CT 06415-0515
       (800) 566-6678

2. Chaselle, Inc.
   (General School Supply Catalogue)
       609 Silver Street, P.O. Box 3004
       Agawam, MA 01001-8004
       (413) 786-9800

3. Creative Crafts
   (New Craft Concepts for Education and Recreation Therapy)
       16 Plains Road, P.O. Box 819
       Essex, CT 06426
       (800) 854-5422

4. Cross Creek Recreational Products, Inc.
   (Independent Activities for the Cognitively Impaired)

RR #1, Box 409A
Amenia, NY 12501
(800) 645-5816

5. Discovery Toys, Inc.
   Martinez, CA 94553
   (800) 426-4777

6. Dover Publications
   31 E. 2nd Street
   Mineola, NY 11501-3582
   (516) 294-7000

7. ElderGames, Inc.
   11710 Hunters Lane
   Rockville, MD 20852
   (800) 637-2604

8. Flag House, Inc.
   (Special Populations—Infant to Adult)
   150 N. MacQuesten Parkway
   Mt. Vernon, NY 10550
   (800) 793-7900

9. Geriatric Resources
   (Sensory Stimulation Products)
   931 S. Semoran Boulevard, #200
   Winter Park, FL 32792
   (800) 359-0390

10. Hammatt Senior Products
    P.O. Box 727
    Mt. Vernon, WA 98273
    (206) 428-5850

11. Lauri, Inc.
    P.O. Box F, Dept. NL
    Phillips-Avon, ME 04966
    (207) 639-2000

12. Nasco Activity Therapy (two addresses)
    901 Janersville Avenue
    Ft. Atkinson, WI 53538-0901
    (414) 563-2446

    1524 Princeton Ave.
    Modesto, CA 95352-3827
    (209) 529-6957

13.   TCA Group, Inc.
        11 Huron Drive
        Natick, MA 01760
14.   World Wide Games
        Colchester, CT 06415
        (203) 537-2325

Bibliography

Adasick, J. 1989. "Humor and the Alzheimer's Patient: The Psychological Basis." *American Journal of Alzheimer's Care and Related Disorders and Research,* July/August, 18–21.

Bailey, E. 1989. "Red on Your Head: Communicating in the Here and Now with Alzheimer's Patients." *American Journal of Alzheimer's Care and Related Disorders and Research,* March/April, 24–27.

Bowman Gray School of Medicine of Wake Forest University. 1994. "Activity Considerations for a Full Day." *Respite Report* (Partners in Caregiving: Dementia Services Program), winter.

Brunette, M. 1988. *The Yankee Caregiver: If You Care for Someone with Alzheimer's Disease.* Augusta, Maine: Kennebec Health Systems.

Cohen, U., and Day, K. 1993. *Contemporary Environments for People with Dementia.* Baltimore: Johns Hopkins University Press.

Dickey, H. 1980. *Reality and the Senses: Activities for Sensory Stimulation.* Buffalo: Potentials Development for Health and Aging Services, Inc.

Dorbacker, B.M. 1994. *Guide for Caregivers.* Gardiner, Maine: Alzheimer's Care Center.

Feil, N. 1952. *Validation Therapy: The Feil Method.* Cleveland: Edward Feil Productions.

Freeman, S. 1987. *Activities and Approaches for Alzheimer's.* St. Simons Island, Ga.: S. Freeman.

Friedman, R., and Tapper, R. 1991. "The Effect of Planned Walking on Communication in Alzheimer's Disease." *Journal of American Geriatric Society* 39: 650–54.

Glynn, N.J. 1992. "The Musical Therapy Assessment Tool in Alzheimer's Patients." *Journal of Gerontological Nursing* 18(1): 3–9.

Gwyther, L. 1985. *Care of Alzheimer's Patients: A Manual for Nursing Home Staff.*

Chicago: American Health Care Association/Alzheimer's Disease and Related Dementias Association.

Hamdy, R.C., et al. 1990. *Alzheimer's Disease: A Handbook for Caregivers.* St. Louis: The C.V. Mosby Co.

Hasselkus, B. 1992. "The Meaning of Activity: Day Care for Persons with A.D." *American Journal of Occupational Therapy* 46(5): 199–206.

Helen, C.R. 1992. *Alzheimer's Disease: Activity Focused Care.* Boston, Mass.: Andover Medical Publishers.

Hirsch, S. 1990. "Dance Therapy in the Service of Dementia." *American Journal of Alzheimer's Care and Related Disorders and Research,* July/August, 26–30.

Hunt, A. 1993. "Humor as a Nursing Intervention." *Cancer Nursing* 16(1): 34–39.

Jacques, J. 1991. "Working with Persons Who Have A.D." *Nursing Homes,* January/February, 16–18.

Kaminsky, M., ed. 1984. *The Uses of Reminiscence.* New York: Haworth Press.

Mace, N.L. 1987. "Principles of Activities for Persons with Dementia." *Physical and Occupational Therapy in Geriatrics* 5(3): 13–27.

Mace, N.L. 1989. *Dementia Care: Patient, Family, and Community.* Baltimore: Johns Hopkins University Press.

Mace, N.L., and Rabins, P.V. 1991. *The 36-Hour Day: A Family Guide to Caring for Persons with Alzheimer's Disease, Related Dementing Illnesses, and Memory Loss in Later Life.* Rev. ed. Baltimore: Johns Hopkins University Press.

Madson, J. 1991. "The Study of Wandering in Persons with Senile Dementia," *American Journal of Alzheimer's Care and Related Disorders and Research,* January/February, 21–24.

McArthur, M.G. 1988. "Exercise as Therapy for the Alzheimer's Patient and Caregiver: Aggressive Action in the Face of an Aggressive Disease." *American Journal of Alzheimer's Care and Related Disorders and Research,* November/December, 36–39.

McConnell, D. 1991. *Rising to the Challenge: Mixed-Level Activity Programming for People with Dementia.* Gardena, Calif.: City of Gardena Publishing.

Meddaugh, D. 1991. "Before Aggression Erupts." *Geriatric Nursing* 12(3): 114–116.

Meyer, D.L., et al. 1990. "A Special Care Home for A.D. and Related Disorders: An 18 Months Progress Report." *American Journal of Alzheimer's Care and Related Disorders and Research,* January/February, 18–23.

Meyer, D.L., et al. 1992. "Effects of a 'Quiet Week' Intervention on Behavior in an Alzheimer's Home." *American Journal of Alzheimer's Care and Related Disorders and Research,* July/August, 2–7.

Namazi, K., and Johnson, B.D. 1992. "The Effects of Environmental Barriers on the Attention Span of Alzheimer's Disease Patients: How Familiar Tasks Can Enhance Concentration in Alzheimer's Disease Patients." *American Journal of Alzheimer's Care and Related Disorders and Research,* January/February, 35–40.

Robinson, V. 1989. *Humor and the Health Professions.* Thorofare, N.J.: Slack.

Sheridan, C. 1987. *Failure-Free Activities for the Alzheimer's Patient.* San Francisco: Cottage Books.

Sloan, P.O., and L.J. Mathew. 1990. "The Therapeutic Environment Screening Scale—An Observational Screening Instrument to Assess the Quality of Nursing Home Environments for Residents with Dementia." *American Journal of Alzheimer's Care and Related Disorders and Research,* November/December, 22–26.

Smith, B.B. 1992. "Treatment of Dementia: Healing through Cultural Arts." *Pride Institute Journal of Long Term Care* 2(3): 37–45.

Teri, L., and Logsdon, R.G. 1991. "Identifying Pleasant Activities for A.D. Patients: The Pleasant Events Schedule." *Gerontologist* 31(1): 124–27.

Thaws, V., et al. 1992. *Now What?: A Handbook of Activities for Adult Day Programs.* Winston-Salem: Bowman Gray School of Medicine of Wake Forest University.

Thornbury, J.M. 1992. "Cognitive Performance on Piagetian Tasks by A.D. Patients." *Research in Nursing and Health* 15: 16–21.

Thornbury, J.M. 1993. "The Use of Piaget's theory in A.D." *American Journal of Alzheimer's Care and Related Disorders and Research,* July/August, 16–21.

Whitcomb, J.B. 1989. "Thanks for the Memory." *American Journal of Alzheimer's Care and Related Disorders and Research,* July/August, 22–23.

Whitcomb, J.B. 1993. "The Way to Go Home: Creating Comfort through Therapeutic Music and Milieu." *American Journal of Alzheimer's Care and Related Disorders and Research,* November/December, 1–10.

Whitlatch, A.M., Meddaugh, D.K., and Langhout, K.J. 1992. "Religiosity among Alzheimer's Disease Caregivers." *American Journal of Alzheimer's Care and Related Disorders and Research,* November/December, 11–19.

Zgola, J. 1987. *Doing Things: A Guide to Programming Activities for Persons with Alzheimer's Disease and Related Disorders.* Baltimore: Johns Hopkins University Press.

Zgola, J. 1988. "I Can Tell You about That." *American Journal of Alzheimer's Care and Related Disorders and Research,* July/August, 17–22.

Index